Problem Based
Cardiology Cases

Problem Based Cardiology Cases

ATIFUR RAHMAN, MBBS, FRACP, FCSANZ
Clinical Director-CCU, Gold Coast University Hospital, Australia
Associate Professor, Griffith University School of Medicine
Honorary Adjunct Associate Professor, Faculty of Health Sciences and Medicine at Bond
    University

SIMON O'CONNOR, FRACP, DDU, FCSANZ
Cardiologist, The Canberra Hospital, Australia
Clinical Senior Lecturer, Australian National University Medical School, Canberra, ACT,
    Australia

ELSEVIER

Elsevier Australia. ACN 001 002 357
(a division of Reed International Books Australia Pty Ltd)
Tower 1, 475 Victoria Avenue, Chatswood, NSW 2067

ISBN: 978-0-7295-4375-0

Notice

Practitioners and researchers must always rely on their own experience and knowledge in evaluating and using any information, methods, compounds or experiments described herein. Because of rapid advances in the medical sciences, in particular, independent verification of diagnoses and drug dosages should be made. To the fullest extent of the law, no responsibility is assumed by Elsevier, authors, editors or contributors for any injury and/or damage to persons or property as a matter of products liability, negligence or otherwise, or from any use or operation of any methods, products, instructions, or ideas contained in the material herein.

National Library of Australia Cataloguing-in-Publication Data

A catalogue record for this
book is available from the
National Library of Australia

Content Strategist: Larissa Norrie
Content Project Manager: Shivani Pal
Edited by Chris Wyard
Proof read by Tim learner
Cover by Georgette Hall
Index by Innodata
Typeset by Toppan Best-set Premedia Limited
Printed in 1010 Printing International Limited

Last digit is the print number: 9 8 7 6 5 4 3 2 1

Acknowledgements

We are very grateful for the help that many people have given us in the preparation of this book. Suggestions, comments and technical assistance have come from many colleagues.

In particular, we wish to thank:

Suzanna Palmer Latona and Dr David Liu, who have drawn some of the figures;

Dr Ian Agahari, Dr Nasser Essack, Dr Hasan Shohag, Michael Trikilis, Luke Shanahan and our hard-working registrars, Dr Rowena Solayar and Dr Farah Najib, who helped in finding some of the clinical images and ECGs;

Cardiology Today and the *Australian Journal of General Practice* (formerly *Australian Family Physician*) – parts of some of the chapters and some images first appeared in these journals and are used with permission;

Some medical images are used with the permission of the Gold Coast Hospital Health Service and The Canberra Hospital.

Foreword

For an Obstetrician, the world of cardiology may be viewed both as mystical, holding special knowledge of the powers of the heart and life itself, and commanding in its strong evidence-based and rigorous approach to problem solving. This book portrays both sides of this speciality and importantly makes this expertise accessible to all aspirational learners in this field.

As often happens it is the personal experience that can bring us to a greater understanding and appreciation of the value of 'expert' and of contemporary evidence based practice, as it did for me recently. My experience also brought with it the added respect for the value of team work, professionalism and respect that ultimately results in high quality and safe clinical care.

In educational terms this book assists the readers in that all-important development from novice to expert.

It is impossible to replicate the quantum of case load learning of the authors overnight but by providing guiding principles, simulation and a problem-based approach the reader can rapidly develop their own case portfolio on that path to expert.

While I commend this book to you, we can be assured that with the fast pace of technological and scientific advancements in this field much of this text will be relegated to history, replaced with even better evidence and better and safer management. And what a good thing that is.

Professor Judy Searle, BMBS FRANZCOG(ret)
MD GDPH GAICD
Foundation Dean, School of Medicine, Griffith University

Preface

No medical specialty has changed more profoundly in the last 20 years than cardiology and, in the view of cardiologists, no specialty is more important. There is no doubt that all cardiologists feel that our ability to look after our patients has improved dramatically over this period. This is probably most evident to us in our management of acute coronary syndromes. Not only does early intervention for these patients improve mortality, but also what used to be common and disabling complications of myocardial infarction are now quite rare. Similar improvements have occurred in the management of heart failure and arrhythmias. Management of valvular heart disease, once always a matter of surgical intervention, is increasingly being undertaken by cardiologists.

In no other area of medicine have changes in practice been so dependent on clinical trials and the use of evidence of the effectiveness, or otherwise, of treatment. New evidence and, as a result, new guidelines for treatment appear constantly.

History taking, physical examination and sensible use of investigations are the basis of all clinical medicine. In this book we have tried to provide a grounding in history taking and examination and have used clinical examples to illustrate important problems in cardiology that clinicians face regularly. There is no substitute for seeing patients in the wards and gaining experience in clinical cardiology, but a case-based approach to learning and decision making complements learning in the wards.

We hope this book will be found useful by senior medical students as they begin to learn about modern cardiology and by general practitioners who want to bring their cardiology practice up to date. Basic physician trainees should also find help here in their FRACP exam preparation. Finally, cardiology and coronary care nurses and technicians may be able to use it to improve their understanding of cardiology practice.

Because of the importance of evidence-based practice in cardiology and the constant new information from clinical trials and updating of guidelines, we have tried to use the latest information and available guidelines. References to trials and guidelines are provided throughout the book.

All efforts have been made to ensure the information given is current and correct but we take responsibility for any errors and of course would be grateful for any comments or corrections from readers.

Our hope is that this book will help bring some of the excitement and satisfaction that modern treatment of cardiology patients has brought to us to many other clinicians.

Atifur Rahman & Simon O'Connor
Gold Coast & Canberra, July 2020

Contents

CHAPTER 1

The Cardiovascular Examination

KEY POINTS

- The cardiovascular examination lends itself to a systematic approach.
- The examination should be thorough but should be directed by the history to areas likely to be relevant.
- Certain cardiovascular signs are quite sensitive and specific.
- When the examination is well performed, many unnecessary investigations can be avoided.

CASE 1 SCENARIO: TARA WITH DYSPNOEA

34-year-old Tara was referred to the hospital by her general practitioner. She presented with increasing dyspnoea for the last 2 weeks. She has found it difficult to lie flat in bed and has been waking up frequently feeling breathless. She also has a dry cough and has felt extremely tired for weeks. She also has high fever with a shake. She is an intravenous drug user and her general practitioner (GP) found a loud murmur on auscultation.

Please examine the cardiovascular system.

The cardiovascular system should be examined in all patients who present with cardiac symptoms. A routine for this examination should be very familiar to students and registrars.

The history should help to direct the examination. For patients with possible heart failure there are certain important signs that support the diagnosis.

AN OUTLINE OF THE CARDIOVASCULAR EXAMINATION

1. Make sure the patient is positioned at 45 degrees and that the chest and neck are fully exposed. For a woman, the requirements of modesty dictate that you cover her breasts with a towel or loose garment.
2. While standing back, inspect for the appearance of Marfan, Turner or Down syndrome. Also look for dyspnoea and cyanosis. It is also worth looking at the neck from a distance. Big v waves are sometimes more obvious from a distance
3. Pick up the patient's hand. Feel the radial pulse. Inspect the patient's hands for clubbing. Demonstrate Schamroth's sign (Fig. 1.1). If there is no clubbing, opposition of the index finger (nail to nail) demonstrates a diamond shape; in clubbing this space is lost. Also look for the peripheral stigmata of infective endocarditis. Splinter haemorrhages are common (and are usually caused by trauma), whereas Osler's nodes and Janeway lesions (Fig. 1.2) are rare. Look quickly, but carefully, at each nail bed, otherwise it is easy to miss key signs. Note the presence of an intravenous cannula and, if an infusion is running, look at the bag to see what it is. There will usually be a peripheral or central line in situ if the patient is being treated for infective endocarditis. Note any tendon xanthomata (type II hyperlipidaemia).
4. The pulse at the wrist should be timed for rate and rhythm. Pulse character is poorly assessed here. This is also the time to feel for radiofemoral delay (which occurs in coarctation of the aorta) and radial–radial inequality.
5. Next inspect the face. Look at the eyes briefly for jaundice (valve haemolysis) and xanthelasma (type II or III hyperlipidaemia) (Fig. 1.3). You may also notice the classic 'mitral facies' (owing to dilation of malar capillaries associated with severe mitral stenosis and caused by pulmonary hypertension and a low cardiac output). Then inspect the mouth using a torch for a high-arched palate (Marfan syndrome and the possibility of aortic regurgitation and mitral valve prolapse), petechiae and the state of dentition (endocarditis). Look at the tongue or lips for central cyanosis.

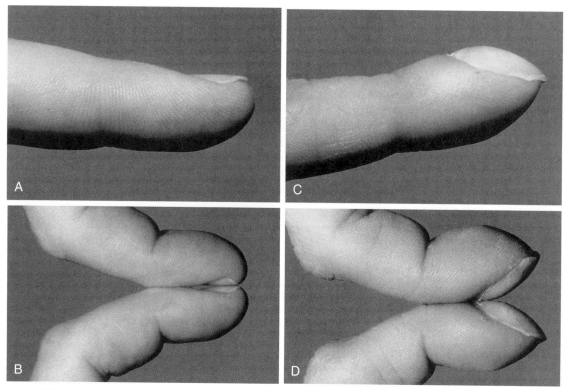

FIG. 1.1 Lateral views of the index finger and Schamroth's sign in a healthy individual **(A** and **B)**, and in an individual with severe clubbing **(C** and **D)**. (From Taussig LM, Landau LI. *Pediatric respiratory medicine*. 2nd ed, Fig. 10-3. Mosby, Elsevier, 2008, with permission.)

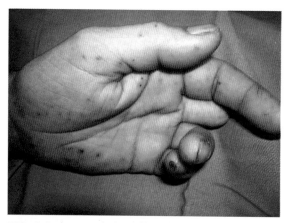

FIG. 1.2 Janeway lesions. (Based on Mandell GL, Bennett JA, Dolin R. *Mandell, Douglas, and Bennett's principles and practice of infectious diseases*. 7th ed, Fig 195-15. Churchill Livingstone, Elsevier, 2009, with permission.)

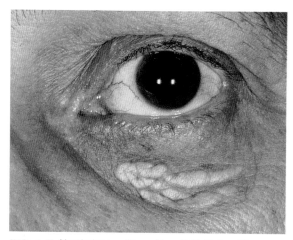

FIG. 1.3 Xanthelasma. (From Yanoff M, Duker JS. *Ophthalmology*. 3rd ed. Fig. 12-9-18. Mosby, Elsevier, 2008, with permission.)

BOX 1.1
Jugular Venous Pressure (JVP)

CAUSES OF AN ELEVATED CENTRAL VENOUS PRESSURE (CVP)

Right ventricular failure

Tricuspid stenosis or regurgitation

Pericardial effusion or constrictive pericarditis

Superior vena caval obstruction

Fluid overload

Hyperdynamic circulation

WAVE FORM
Causes of a Dominant a Wave

Tricuspid stenosis (also causing a slow **y** descent)

Pulmonary stenosis

Pulmonary hypertension

Causes of Cannon a Waves

Complete heart block

Paroxysmal nodal tachycardia with retrograde atrial conduction

Ventricular tachycardia with retrograde atrial conduction or atrioventricular dissociation

Causes of a Dominant v Wave

Tricuspid regurgitation

x Descent

Absent: atrial fibrillation

Exaggerated: acute cardiac tamponade, constrictive pericarditis

y Descent

Sharp: severe tricuspid regurgitation, constrictive pericarditis

Slow: tricuspid stenosis, right atrial myxoma

(From Talley N, O'Connor S, *Clinical examination*. 8th ed, vol. 1, p. 92, with permission.)

6. The neck is very important, so take time to examine here. The jugular venous pressure (JVP) must be assessed for height and character (see Box 1.1 and Fig. 1.4). Use the right internal jugular vein to assess this. Normally the JVP falls with inspiration; elevation during inspiration is called Kussmaul's sign.

7. Now feel each carotid pulse separately. Assess the pulse character (see Box 1.1).

8. Proceed to the chest. Look *everywhere* for scars. Previous mitral valvotomy may have been performed

by a submammary or lateral thoracotomy approach. These patients slowly redevelop mitral stenosis over many years. Inspect for deformity, the site of the apex beat and visible pulsations. Do not forget about pacemaker and cardioverter–defibrillator boxes (see Fig. 1.4).

9. Palpate for the apex beat position. Count down the correct number of intercostal spaces. The normal position is the fifth intercostal space, 1 cm medial to the midclavicular line. The character of the apex beat is important. There are a number of types.

    a. A *pressure-loaded* (hyperdynamic, systolic-overloaded) apex beat is a forceful and sustained impulse (e.g. in aortic stenosis, hypertension).

    b. A *volume-loaded* (hyperkinetic, diastolic-overloaded) apex beat is a forceful but unsustained impulse (e.g. in aortic regurgitation, mitral regurgitation).

10. Don't miss the tapping apex beat of mitral stenosis (a palpable first heart sound) or the dyskinetic apex beat caused by a previous large myocardial infarction. The double or triple apical impulse in hypertrophic cardiomyopathy is very important too. Feel also for an apical thrill and time it.

11. Palpate with the heel of your hand for a left parasternal impulse, which indicates right ventricular hypertrophy or left atrial enlargement. Feel at the base of the heart for a palpable pulmonary component of the second heart sound (P2) and aortic thrills. Percussion is usually unnecessary.

12. Auscultation begins with listening in the mitral area with both the bell and the diaphragm. Spend most time here. Listen for each component of the cardiac cycle separately. Identify the first and second heart sounds (see Fig. 1.4) and decide whether they are of normal intensity and whether they are split. Now listen for extra heart or prosthetic heart sounds and murmurs. Mechanical valves include bileaflet, ball-in-cage and tilting-disc types. Ball-in-cage valves have a sharp opening sound and may rattle. Tilting-disc valves have soft opening sounds and sharp closing sounds.

13. Repeat the approach at the left sternal edge and then at the base of the heart (aortic and pulmonary areas). Time each part of the cycle with the carotid pulse. Listen below the left clavicle for a patent ductus arteriosus murmur, which may be audible here and nowhere else.

14. It is now time to reposition the patient, first in the left lateral position. Again feel the apex beat for character (particularly tapping). Auscultate carefully for mitral stenosis with the bell. Next sit

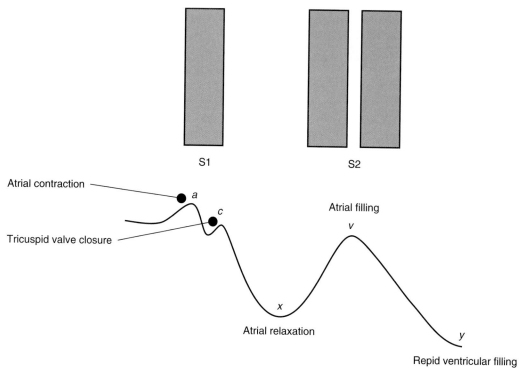

FIG. 1.4 The JVP and its relationship to the first (S1) and second (S2) heart sounds. (From Talley N, O'Connor S, *Examination medicine.* 8th ed, p. 394, fig 16.4, with permission.)

the patient forward and feel for thrills (with the patient in full expiration) at the left sternal edge and base. Then listen in those areas, particularly for aortic regurgitation.

15. Dynamic auscultation should always be done if there is any doubt about the diagnosis. The Valsalva manoeuvre should be performed whenever there is a systolic murmur, otherwise hypertrophic cardiomyopathy is easily missed

16. The patient is now sitting up. Percuss the back quickly to exclude a pleural effusion (e.g. due to left ventricular failure) and auscultate for inspiratory crackles (left ventricular failure). If there is radiofemoral delay, also listen for a coarctation murmur here. Feel for sacral oedema and note any back deformity (ankylosing spondylitis is associated with aortic regurgitation).

17. Next lay the patient flat and examine the abdomen for hepatomegaly (e.g. as a result of right ventricular failure) and a pulsatile liver (tricuspid regurgitation). Perform the hepatojugular reflux test. Press over the upper abdomen for 15 seconds or so and watch for a rise in the JVP. This is a reliable sign of heart failure. Feel for splenomegaly (endocarditis) and an aortic aneurysm. Palpate both femoral arteries. Then examine all the peripheral pulses. Look particularly for peripheral oedema, clubbing of the toes, Achilles tendon xanthomata (Fig. 1.5), signs of peripheral vascular disease and the stigmata of infective endocarditis.

18. The results of the urine analysis (haematuria) and the temperature chart (fever) and examination of the fundi (for Roth's spots (Fig. 1.6)) are necessary if endocarditis is a possibility. The fundi should also be examined for hypertensive changes.

Certain symptoms and signs are quite sensitive and specific for the diagnosis of heart failure. When a patient presents with possible heart failure (often with problems with dyspnoea) the history and examination will often help with the diagnosis and in distinguishing heart failure from other causes of breathlessness (Box 1.2).

LEFT VENTRICULAR FAILURE (LVF)

• **Symptoms:** exertional dyspnoea, orthopnoea, paroxysmal nocturnal dyspnoea.

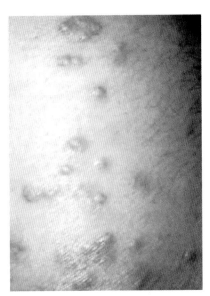

FIG. 1.5 Xanthomata. (From Durrington P. Dyslipidaemia, *Lancet* 2003;362:717–31, with permission.)

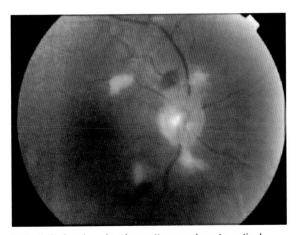

FIG. 1.6 A retina showing cotton wool spots, retinal haemorrhage and Roth's spot in a septic bacteraemic cancer patient. (From Celik I, Cihangiroflu M, Yilmaz T. The prevalence of bacteraemia-related retinal lesions in seriously ill patients. *J Infect* 2006;52(2):97–104, Fig. 1, with permission.)

- **General signs:** tachypnoea, due to raised pulmonary pressures; central cyanosis, due to pulmonary oedema; Cheyne–Stokes breathing especially in sedated elderly patients; peripheral cyanosis, due to low cardiac output; hypotension, due to low cardiac output; cardiac cachexia.

BOX 1.2
Findings That Favour Heart Failure as the Cause of Dyspnoea

- History of myocardial infarction
- No wheeze
- Paroxysmal nocturnal dyspnoea (PND)[a]
- Orthopnoea
- Abnormal apex beat
- Third heart sound (S3)
- Mitral regurgitant murmur
- Early and mid-inspiratory crackles
- Cough only on lying down

[a]*Paroxysmal nocturnal dyspnoea* (PND) is a sensation of shortness of breath that awakens the patient, often after 1 or 2 hours of sleep, and is usually relieved in the upright position.

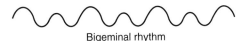

Bigeminal rhythm

FIG. 1.7 Pulsus alternans.

- **Arterial pulse:** sinus tachycardia, due to increased sympathetic tone; low pulse pressure (low cardiac output); pulsus alternans (alternate strong and weak beats) (Fig. 1.7); it is unlike a bigeminal rhythm caused by regular ectopic beats, in that the beats are regular – this is a rare but specific sign of unknown aetiology.
- **Apex beat:** displaced, with dilation of the left ventricle; dyskinetic in anterior myocardial infarction or dilated cardiomyopathy; palpable gallop rhythm. The absence of these signs does not exclude left ventricular failure.
- **Auscultation:** left ventricular S3 (an important sign); functional mitral regurgitation (secondary to valve ring dilation).
- **Lung fields:** signs of pulmonary congestion (basal inspiratory crackles) or pulmonary oedema (crackles and wheezes throughout the lung fields), due to raised venous pressures (increased preload). The typical middle-to-late inspiratory crackles at the lung bases may be absent in chronic, compensated heart failure, and there are many other causes of basal inspiratory crackles. This makes crackles a rather non-specific and insensitive sign of heart failure.
- **Other signs:** abnormal Valsalva response; positive abdominojugular reflux test; right ventricular failure may complicate left ventricular failure, especially if this is severe and chronic.

- **Signs of the underlying or precipitating cause:**
  - *Causes of LVF:* (1) myocardial disease (ischaemic heart disease, cardiomyopathy); (2) volume overload (aortic regurgitation, mitral regurgitation, patent ductus arteriosus); (3) pressure overload (systolic hypertension, aortic stenosis).
  - *Signs of a precipitating cause:* anaemia, thyrotoxicosis, rapid arrhythmia (usually atrial fibrillation). (See Good signs guide 1.1.)

RIGHT VENTRICULAR FAILURE (RVF)

- **Symptoms:** ankle, sacral or abdominal swelling, anorexia, nausea.
- **General signs:** peripheral cyanosis, due to low cardiac output.
- **Arterial pulse:** low volume, due to low cardiac output.
- **Jugular venous pulse:** raised, due to the raised venous pressure (right heart preload); Kussmaul's sign, due to poor right ventricular compliance (e.g. right ventricular myocardial infarction); large v waves (functional tricuspid regurgitation secondary to valve ring dilation).
- **Praecordial palpation:** parasternal impulse (right ventricular heave).
- **Auscultation:** right ventricular S3; pansystolic murmur of functional tricuspid regurgitation (absence of a murmur does not exclude tricuspid regurgitation).
- **Abdomen:** tender hepatomegaly, due to increased venous pressure transmitted via the hepatic veins; pulsatile liver (a useful sign), if tricuspid regurgitation is present.
- **Oedema:** due to sodium and water retention plus raised venous pressure; may be manifested by pitting ankle and sacral oedema, ascites or pleural effusions (small).
- **Signs of the underlying cause:**
  - *Causes of RVF:* (1) chronic obstructive pulmonary disease (most common cause of cor pulmonale); (2) left ventricular failure (severe chronic LVF causes raised pulmonary pressures resulting in secondary right ventricular failure); (3) volume overload (atrial septal defect, primary tricuspid regurgitation); (4) other causes of pressure overload (pulmonary stenosis, idiopathic pulmonary hypertension); (5) myocardial disease (right ventricular myocardial infarction, cardiomyopathy).

GOOD SIGNS GUIDE 1.1
Left Ventricular Failure in a Patient With Dyspnoea

General Signs	LR+	LR−
Heart rate >100 beats per minute at rest	5.5	NS
Abdominojugular reflux test	6.4	0.79
LUNGS		
Crackles	2.8	0.5
CARDIAC EXAMINATION		
JVP elevated	5.1	0.66
S4	NS	NS
Apex displaced lateral to midclavicular line	5.8	NS
S3	11	0.88
Any murmur	2.6	0.81
OTHER FINDINGS		
Oedema	2.3	0.64
Wheezing	0.22	1.3
Ascites	0.33	1.0
THE HISTORY (GOOD SYMPTOMS GUIDE)		
Paroxysmal nocturnal dyspnoea	2.6	0.7
Orthopnoea	2.2	0.65
Dyspnoea on exertion	1.3	0.48
Fatigue and weight gain	1.0	0.99
Previous heart failure	5.8	0.45
Previous myocardial infarction	3.1	0.69
Hypertension	1.4	0.7
COPD	0.81	1.1

COPD=chronic obstructive pulmonary disease; JVP=jugular venous pressure; LR=likelihood ratio; NS=not significant.
(From Talley N, O'Connor S, *Clinical examination medicine.* 8th ed, p. 120, with permission.)

Common Valvular Heart Disease

AORTIC STENOSIS

The normal area of the aortic valve is more than 2 cm^2. Significant narrowing of this valve restricts left ventricular outflow and imposes a pressure load on the left ventricle.

- **Symptoms:** exertional chest pain (50% do not have coronary artery disease), exertional dyspnoea and exertional syncope.

CASE 2 SCENARIO: BILL WITH HEART MURMUR

Mr Bill Reeves is a 78-year-old man who has been booked for a routine colonoscopy because of a family history of carcinoma of the colon. The anaesthetist who examined him told him he had a heart murmur, and that he should put off his colonoscopy and have his heart checked.

Symptoms and Signs
What questions would you ask Bill?

- Always ask general questions about previous cardiac problems and cardiac risk factors.

'Has this murmur ever been picked up before?' People sometimes forget they have been told previously about a problem.

'Have you had any problems with shortness of breath? Is this getting worse?'

'Yes a little.'

'What sort of exercise do you do?'

'I walk my dog regularly and sometimes lately I have a little trouble keeping up because I am short of breath. I think I am getting older faster than she is.'

'Have you had high blood pressure?'

'No.'

'Do you know your cholesterol level?'

'About 6, I think.'

'Is there a history of heart disease in the family?'

'No.'

'Have you had any other problems with your health – kidney trouble, liver trouble, or a stroke?'

'No.'

- Most valve problems lead to dyspnoea when they become severe.

'When you feel breathless, is there any feeling of tightness or discomfort in the chest?'

- Patients with severe AS often describe chest tightness very similar to angina.

'Have you ever blacked out or nearly blacked out during exercise?'

- Patients with very severe AS may experience exertional syncope. The patient thinks he has been more breathless on exertion than he was a year ago and he has noticed a feeling of mild chest tightness when he walks up hills.

What examination would you perform?
- A complete cardiovascular examination is indicated (see Chapter 1).

What signs would you expect to find if he has AS and how would you decide clinically on the severity?
- **General signs:** usually there is nothing remarkable about the general appearance.
- **Pulse:** there may be a plateau or anacrotic pulse, or the pulse may be late peaking (*tardus*) and of small volume (*parvus*).
- **Palpation:** the apex beat is hyperdynamic and may be slightly displaced, with a systolic thrill at the base of the heart (aortic area).
- **Auscultation:** a narrowly split or reversed S2 because of delayed left ventricular ejection; a harsh midsystolic ejection murmur, maximal over the aortic area and extending into the carotid arteries, is characteristic. However, it may be heard widely over the praecordium and extend to the apex. The murmur is loudest with the patient sitting up and in full expiration; associated aortic regurgitation is common; in congenital AS where the valve cusps remain mobile and the dome of the valve comes to a sudden halt, an ejection click may precede the murmur – the ejection click is absent if the valve is calcified or if the stenosis is not at the valve level but above or below it (supra- or subvalvular stenosis).
- **Signs indicating severe AS (Good signs guide 2.1):** valve area less than 1 cm², or valve gradient greater than 50 mmHg; plateau pulse, carotid pulse reduced in force; thrill in the aortic area; length of the murmur and lateness of the peak of the systolic murmur; soft or absent A2; left ventricular failure (very late sign); pressure-loaded apex beat. These signs are not reliable

for distinguishing between moderate and severe disease. It is important to remember that the signs of severity of AS are less reliable in the elderly.[1]
- **Causes of AS:** (1) degenerative calcific AS, particularly in elderly patients; (2) calcific in younger patients, usually on a congenital bicuspid valve; (3) rheumatic.
- **Other types of aortic outflow obstruction are also possible:**
  1. supravalvular obstruction, where there is narrowing of the ascending aorta or a fibrous diaphragm just above the aortic valve – this is rare and may be associated with a characteristic facies (a broad forehead, widely set eyes and a pointed chin); there is a loud A2 and often a thrill in the area of the sternal notch
  2. subvalvular obstruction, where there is a membranous diaphragm or fibrous ridge just below the aortic valve – aortic regurgitation is associated with it and is due to a jet lesion affecting the coronary cusp of the valve
  3. dynamic left ventricular outflow tract obstruction, which may occur in hypertrophic cardiomyopathy – here there may be a double apical impulse. Atrial contraction into a stiff left ventricle may be palpable before the left ventricular impulse (only in the presence of sinus rhythm, of course).

Aortic sclerosis presents in the elderly; there are none of the peripheral signs of AS. The diagnosis implies the absence of a gradient across the aortic valve despite some thickening and a murmur.

You find a harsh ejection systolic murmur that radiates to the carotids and a thrill that is palpable over the base of the heart.

These symptoms and signs suggest severe AS.

Investigations
What investigations would you arrange?
- The echocardiogram is the investigation of choice.
- The chest x-ray may show characteristic abnormalities (valve calcification), but has largely been superseded.
- Cardiac CT scanning is increasingly used in difficult cases. The severity of valve calcification correlates with the severity of the stenosis.

What might you expect to see on his ECG?
- The ECG may be normal, but changes of left ventricular hypertrophy are likely.

What information would you expect from the echocardiogram?
- General information from 2D scanning including left ventricle (LV) systolic function, presence of left

GOOD SIGNS GUIDE 2.1 Severe Aortic Stenosis		
Sign	**LR+**	**LR−**
Delayed carotid upstroke	9.2	0.56
Diminished carotid pulse on palpation	2.0	0.64
Absent or decreased A2	7.5	0.5
Murmur over right clavicle	3.0	0.1
Any systolic murmur	2.6	0
Murmur radiates to the right carotid artery	8.1	0.29

LR = likelihood ratio.

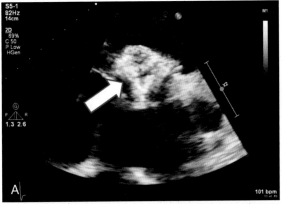

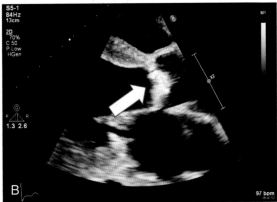

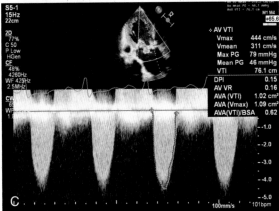

FIG. 2.1 Calcific aortic valve with severe stenosis (white arrow): **(A)** in short-axis view and **(B)** in the parasternal long-axis view. **(C)** Peak systolic velocity across the aortic valve.

ventricle hypertrophy (LVH) and valve morphology (e.g. the extent of calcification, limitation of valve cusp movement, a bicuspid valve) (see Fig. 2.1).

- Doppler measurements of valve gradient and calculation of valve area.
- Table 2.1 shows the European Society of Cardiology (ESC) criteria for the diagnosis of severe AS.[1]

The echocardiogram report is of a heavily calcified valve with a mean gradient of 65 mmHg. The valve area was calculated to be 0.7 cm[2].

There is a mild increase in LV wall thickness consistent with LVH. The ejection fraction is 60% (normal).

Indications for Intervention in Aortic Stenosis
Surgical vs transcatheter aortic valve implantation – what would you advise him should be done?

- This man has severe AS and is symptomatic. He has no contraindications to cardiac surgery. He should be offered surgical aortic valve replacement.

He has heard about valve replacement without surgery and wants to know if he can have that.

- Transcatheter aortic valve implantation (TAVI) is increasingly used for patients with AS. In Australia it is generally reserved for patients who are too unwell to have surgical treatment. The indications for TAVI are widening, however. In many parts of Europe he would be offered TAVI if that were his preference.
- It might be of some consolation to him to point out that the results of surgical valve replacement for someone without co-morbidities are excellent.
- His calculated EuroSCORE (see Table 2.2) would indicate <2% surgical mortality.[2]
- The medium- and long-term data for TAVI in patients <75 years are not yet available. Table 2.2 shows some of the criteria used to help in the choice of TAVI or surgical aortic valve replacement (SAVR).

He asks if there is any alternative to valve replacement.

- No medical treatment has been shown to improve the outcome for patients with AS. Statins have not been shown to alter the natural history of the disease.[1]

TABLE 2.1
ESC Criteria for the Diagnosis of Severe Aortic Stenosis

Criteria	
Clinical criteria	Typical symptoms without other explanation Age >70
Qualitative imaging data	LV hypertrophy (but consider previous hypertension as a possible cause) Reduced longitudinal LV function without other cause
Quantitative data	Mean gradient 30–40 mmHg Aortic valve area ≤0.8 cm² Calcium score by multislice CT: Severe AS very likely: men ≥3000; women ≥1600 Severe AS likely; men ≥2000, women ≥1200 Severe AS unlikely; men <1600; women <800

AS = aortic stenosis; LV = left ventricular.
(Modified from Baumgartner H, Falk V, Bax J, De Bonis M, Hamm C, Holm P, et al. 2017 ESC/EACTS guidelines for the management of valvular heart disease. *Eur Heart J* 2017;38(36):2757, with permission.)

Treatment with diuretics, control of blood pressure and maintenance of sinus rhythm can help with symptoms.

Should he defer his colonoscopy?
- Non-urgent colonoscopy should be deferred.

Are any other investigations indicated?
- Coronary angiography is indicated. Fifty percent of these patients have significant coronary disease and need coronary artery bypass grafting at the time of their valve replacement.

Should he have a bioprosthetic or mechanical valve?
- Patients who are older than 60 or 65 years almost always have a bioprosthetic valve. The longevity of modern bovine pericardial valves is 15–20 years in the aortic position. The advantage of indefinite longevity of mechanical valves is outweighed by the long-term risks of anticoagulation with warfarin.
- The patient must make an informed choice about the type of valve, taking into consideration the possible need for reoperation (or TAVI) following degeneration of a bioprosthesis and the risks of anticoagulation. Remember that the novel oral anticoagulants are contraindicated for patients with mechanical valves.[3,4]

The coronary angiogram shows a 75% proximal left anterior descending artery (LAD) stenosis. He goes on to have a bioprosthetic aortic valve replacement and left internal mammary bypass graft (LIMA) to the LAD.

Apart from a 3-hour episode of atrial fibrillation on the second postoperative day, there are no complications. He spends 6 days in hospital.

Long-Term Management and Follow-Up
What long-term medications are indicated?
- Aspirin is recommended for all bioprosthetic valve patients for 3 months, and indefinitely for people who have had coronary artery bypass surgery. There is no evidence to support longer use of aspirin for patients with a bioprosthetic valve who do not have coronary disease, but it is often prescribed.[1]
- His cholesterol was elevated and he has coronary disease; he should be prescribed a statin.

How should he be followed up?
The ESC guidelines suggest a baseline echocardiogram at about 4 weeks. This will enable:
- the valve morphology to be examined
- a paravalvular leak to be detected (not significant if mild)
- the valve gradient to be measured (should be less than 20 mmHg if the valve is correctly sized)
- assessment of LV function (very occasionally impaired following surgery as a result of inadequate cardioplegia or a perioperative infarct – graft failure).

Annual echocardiographic assessment is then suggested.

He asks when he can get back to normal activities.
- Most patients have very little pain from their sternal wounds but should avoid heavy lifting and golf swings for about 6 weeks.
- Patients will normally be enrolled in a cardiac rehabilitation program where they can begin supervised exercises and have their sternal healing monitored. These have been shown to help accelerate the return to normal activities and work for patients.

MITRAL REGURGITATION
Mitral regurgitation (MR) is the second most common abnormality after AS in developed countries.

TABLE 2.2
Criteria Used to Help in the Choice of Transcatheter Aortic Valve Implantation or Surgical Aortic Valve Replacement

	Favours TAVI	Favours SAVR
CLINICAL		
EuroSCORE >4%[a]	+	
EuroSCORE <4%		+
Presence of severe co-morbidity (not reflected in score)	+	
Age <75		+
Age >75	+	
Previous cardiac surgery	+	
Frailty	+	
Restricted mobility that will impair recovery	+	
Possible endocarditis		+
ANATOMY		
Favourable transfemoral access for TAVI	+	
Unfavourable access for TAVI, e.g. severe peripheral vascular disease		+
Previous chest irradiation	+	
Heavily calcified aortic wall	+	
Previous bypass grafts that are patent	+	
Severe chest wall deformity	+	
Short distance between coronary ostia and aortic valve annulus		+
Aortic root morphology unfavourable for TAVI		+
Bicuspid valve, heavy calcification, aortic regurgitation		+
LV or aortic thrombus		+
OTHER CARDIAC CONDITIONS		
Severe coronary disease requiring revascularisation		+
Severe mitral or tricuspid valve disease		+
Aneurysm of the ascending aorta		+

[a]European System for Cardiac Operative Risk Evaluation; calculator: http://www.euroscore.org/calge.html.
LV=left ventricular; SAVR=surgical aortic valve replacement; TAVI=transcatheter aortic valve implantation.
(Modified from Baumgartner H, Falk V, Bax J, De Bonis M, Hamm C, Holm P, et al. 2017 ESC/EACTS guidelines for the management of valvular heart disease. *Eur Heart J* 2017;38(36):2757, with permission.)

CASE 3 SCENARIO: MRS AB WITH EXERTIONAL DYSPNOEA

Mrs AB, a 58-year-old woman, presents with gradually increasing exertional dyspnoea over 18 months. She thinks this may be a result of some weight gain and loss of fitness but is distressed that she cannot keep up with her walking group. She has had no orthopnoea or paroxysmal dyspnoea.

Symptoms and Signs
What questions would you ask Mrs AB?

- As always, ask general questions about previous cardiac problems and cardiac risk factors.
  'Has this murmur ever been picked up before?'
  People sometimes forget they have been told previously about a problem.
  She was told 15 years ago that she might have a 'floppy valve' but cannot remember whether she had

any tests done. She was told she should have antibiotic prophylaxis before dental and surgical procedures.

'Have you had any problems with shortness of breath? Is this getting worse?'

'I think so. I can't keep up with my walking group anymore. I think I am just unfit and getting older but I want to make sure my heart is all right.'

'Have you been short of breath at night and had to sleep sitting up on pillows?' (orthopnoea)

Have you ever woken at night gasping for breath?' (paroxysmal nocturnal dyspnoea, or PND)

'No.'

'Have you had high blood pressure?'

'Yes.'

'Have you been treated for that?'

'Yes I take ramipril tablets – 5 mg I think.'

'Has the blood pressure been under good control?'

'My doctor always seems happy with it.'

'Do you know your cholesterol level?'

'About 6, I think.'

'Is there a history of heart disease in the family?'

'My father had a heart attack when he was about 80.'

'Have you had any other problems with your health – kidney trouble, liver trouble, a stroke?'

'No.'

Most valve problems lead to dyspnoea when they become severe.

What examination would you perform?
- A complete cardiovascular examination is indicated as always (see Chapter 1).

What signs would you expect to find if she has MR, and how would you decide clinically on the severity?
A regurgitant mitral valve allows part of the left ventricular stroke volume to regurgitate into the left atrium, imposing a volume load on both the left atrium and the left ventricle.

General signs of severe MR: tachypnoea
- **Pulse:** normal, or sharp upstroke due to rapid left ventricular decompression; atrial fibrillation is relatively common.
- **Palpation:** the apex beat may be displaced, diffuse and hyperdynamic in cases of severe MR; a pansystolic thrill is occasionally present at the apex (very severe MR); a parasternal impulse may be present (due to left atrial enlargement behind the right ventricle – the left atrium is often larger in MR than in mitral stenosis and can be enormous).

- **Auscultation:** soft or absent S1 (by the end of diastole, atrial and ventricular pressures have equalised and the valve cusps have drifted back together); sometimes a left ventricular S3, which is due to rapid left ventricular filling in early diastole and, when soft, does not imply severe regurgitation; pansystolic murmur maximal at the apex and usually radiating towards the axilla
- **Mitral valve prolapse:** this syndrome can cause a systolic murmur or click, or both, at the apex. The presence of the murmur indicates that there is some MR present.
- **Auscultation:** there may be a midsystolic click followed by a middle and late systolic murmur that extends to the second heart sound. It often has a blowing quality. There may, however, be a click and no murmur (suggests little or no regurgitation) or a typical murmur without an audible click. The murmur may be pansystolic.
- **Dynamic auscultation:** murmur and click occur earlier and may become louder with the Valsalva manoeuvre and with standing (unlike the ejection click of aortic or pulmonary stenosis), but with squatting and isometric exercise both murmur and click occur later and may become softer.
- **Causes of mitral valve prolapse:**
  1. myxomatous degeneration of the mitral valve tissue – it is very common, especially in women; the severity may increase with age, particularly in men, so that significant MR may supervene
  2. it may be associated with atrial septal defect (secundum), hypertrophic cardiomyopathy or Marfan syndrome.
- **Signs indicating severe chronic MR:** small-volume pulse; enlarged left ventricle; loud S3; soft S1; A2 is early, because rapid left ventricular decompression into the left atrium causes the aortic valve to close early; early diastolic rumble; signs of pulmonary hypertension; signs of left ventricular failure.

  Severe MR is associated with raised pulmonary artery pressures and tricuspid regurgitation. There may be i waves visible in the neck and a pulsatile liver – signs of TR.

Note: Remember all the causes of MR.
- **Causes of chronic MR:**
  1. mitral valve prolapse
  2. 'degenerative' – associated with ageing
  3. rheumatic
  4. papillary muscle dysfunction, due to left ventricular failure or ischaemia

5. cardiomyopathy – hypertrophic, dilated or restrictive cardiomyopathy
6. connective tissue disease (e.g. Marfan syndrome, rheumatoid arthritis, ankylosing spondylitis)
7. congenital (e.g. atrioventricular canal defect).

The examination reveals:
- no dyspnoea at rest
- pulse rate 85 and regular, normal character
- blood pressure 125/75
- JVP – visible v waves
- apex beat – displaced 1 cm from midaxillary line
- 3/6 middle and late systolic murmur at the apex
- no S3
- chest clear to auscultation
- liver pulsatile.

What signs suggest the MR is severe?
- The displaced apex beat
- Signs of tricuspid regurgitation suggesting raised pulmonary artery pressures and therefore severe MR.

Investigations
What investigations will be helpful?
The echocardiogram will give the information needed for the assessment (**Fig. 2.2**):
- severity (see Table 2.3)
- the mechanism of the regurgitation
- signs of LV dysfunction (including the ejection fraction)
- the left atrial size
- the presence of pulmonary hypertension

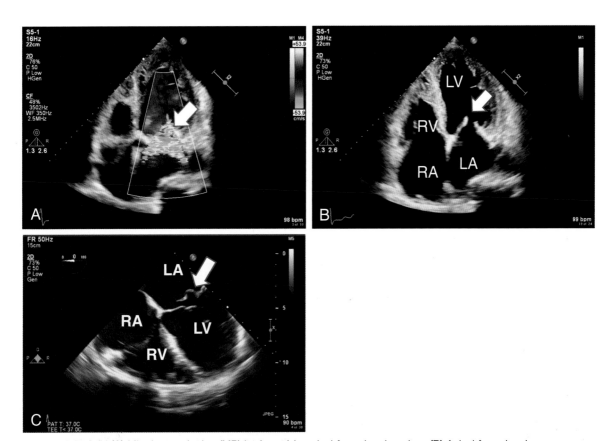

FIG. 2.2 **(A)** Mitral regurgitation (MR) jet (arrow) in apical four-chamber view. **(B)** Apical four-chamber view showing left ventricle (LV), left atrium (LA) right ventricle (RV) and right atrium (RA). Arrow represents the mitral valve. **(C)** Severe MR due to flail posterior mitral valve leaflet (arrow) in a different patient.

TABLE 2.3
ESC Criteria for the Definition of Severe Mitral Regurgitation

QUALITATIVE	
Valve morphology	Flail leaflet, ruptured papillary muscle, large coaptation defect
Colour flow regurgitant jet	Very large central jet or eccentric jet adhering, swirling and reaching the posterior wall of the LA
Continuous wave signal of jet	Dense/triangular
Other	Large-flow convergence zone
SEMIQUANTITATIVE	
Width of vena contracta	>7 mm
Upstream vein flow	Systolic pulmonary vein reversal
Inflow	E-wave dominant >1.5 m/s
QUANTITATIVE	
Effective regurgitant orifice area (mm²)	>40 (primary MR); >20 (secondary MR)
Regurgitant volume (mL/beat)	>60 (primary MR); >30 (secondary MR)
Enlargement of chambers	LV, LA

LA=left atrium; LV=left ventricular; MR=mitral regurgitation.
(From Baumgartner H, Falk V, Bax J, De Bonis M, Hamm C, Holm P, et al. 2017 ESC/EACTS guidelines for the management of valvular heart disease. *Eur Heart J* 2017;38(36): 2757, with permission.)

- suitability for valve repair.

Sometimes, transoesophageal echo is indicated if image quality is poor, so that the morphology of the valve and the possibility of valve repair can be assessed.

The echocardiogram shows (Fig. 2.3):
- moderate left ventricular dilation
- left atrial dilation
- severe prolapse of the posterior mitral valve leaflet
- a vena contracta of 8 mm
- a large regurgitant eccentric jet extending to the posterior wall of the left atrium
- reversal of flow in the pulmonary veins
- mild tricuspid regurgitation and mildly elevated right ventricular systolic pressure
- an ejection fraction of 55%

Indications for Intervention in Mitral Regurgitation
What would you recommend to the patient?
Surgery is recommended (ESC guidelines, p. 2759) for symptomatic patients with severe MR.[5,6]

What are the surgical options?
These are listed in Box 2.1.

What other investigations are indicated before she has surgery?
Cardiac catheterisation is required for patients older than 30 years who need valve surgery. This is to image the coronary arteries. Coronary artery bypass grafting is performed at the same time as valve surgery if significant coronary disease (lesions >70%) is detected.

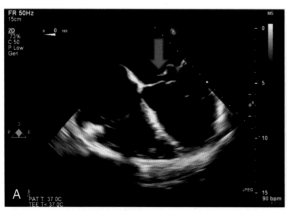
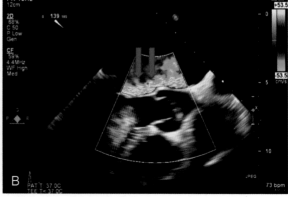

FIG. 2.3 **(A)** Transoesophageal echocardiography (TOE) showing prolapsed posterior mitral valve leaflet (single arrow), with **(B)** eccentric mitral regurgitation (double arrow).

BOX 2.1
Mitral Valve Repair: ESC Indications for Intervention in Severe Primary Mitral Regurgitation

- **Class I Level C:** mitral valve repair should be the preferred technique when the results are expected to be durable.
- **Class I level B:** surgery is indicated in symptomatic patients with LVEF >30%.
- **Class I level B:** surgery is indicated in asymptomatic patients with LV dysfunction (LVESD ≥45 mm and/or LVEF ≤60%).
- **Class IIa level B:** surgery should be considered in asymptomatic patients with preserved LV function (LVESD <45 mm and LVEF >60%) and atrial fibrillation secondary to mitral regurgitation or pulmonary hypertension (systolic pulmonary pressure at rest >50 mmHg).
- **Class IIa level C:** surgery should be considered in asymptomatic patients with preserved LVEF (>60%) and LVESD 40–44 mm when a durable repair is likely, surgical risk is low, the repair is performed in a heart valve centre and at least one of the following findings is present:

- flail leaflet, or
- presence of significant LA dilation (volume index ≥60 mL/m² BSA) in sinus rhythm.
- **Class IIa Level C:** mitral valve repair should be considered in symptomatic patients with severe LV dysfunction (LVEF <30% and/or LVESD >55 mm) refractory to medical therapy when the likelihood of successful repair is high and co-morbidity is low.
- **Class IIb Level C:** mitral valve replacement may be considered in symptomatic patients with severe LV dysfunction (LVEF <30% and/or LVESD >55 mm) refractory to medical therapy when the likelihood of successful repair is low and co-morbidity is low.
- **Class IIb Level C:** percutaneous edge-to-edge procedure may be considered in patients with symptomatic severe primary mitral regurgitation who fulfil the echocardiographic criteria of eligibility and are judged inoperable or at high surgical risk by the heart team, avoiding futility.

BSA=body surface area; LA=left atrial; LV=left ventricular; LVEF=left ventricular ejection fraction; LVESD=left ventricular end-systolic diameter.
(Based on Baumgartner H, Falk V, Bax J, De Bonis M, Hamm C, Holm P, et al. 2017 ESC/EACTS guidelines for the management of valvular heart disease. *Eur Heart J* 2017;38(36):2739–86.

What are the disadvantages of mitral valve replacement compared with repair?

Repair of the valve preserves papillary muscle function. Successful repair operations give a very durable result with low probability of the need for further surgery. Long-term anticoagulation with warfarin is not required. Patients in atrial fibrillation can be treated with a novel oral anticoagulant drug. The surgery can be technically difficult and should be performed by a surgeon experienced in valve repair.

Tissue mitral valve replacement is a simpler operation but the durability of tissue valves in the mitral position is variable and failure within 5–7 years can occur.

Mechanical mitral valve replacement gives a durable result but anticoagulation with warfarin is required, with target international normalised ratio (INR) readings in the high range of 3–3.5. The thrombotic risk associated with mechanical mitral valves is higher than that with aortic valves and the bleeding risk with the higher-target INR is also higher.

The coronary angiogram shows minimal coronary disease. Mrs AB has mitral valve repair surgery. She is in hospital for 6 days. There is a brief episode of postoperative atrial fibrillation.

She is referred to a cardiac rehabilitation course and rapidly regains her confidence and previous exercise ability. Within 5 weeks she feels she has an improved exercise tolerance.

Long-Term Management and Follow-Up
What continuing medications and follow-up are indicated?

A routine echocardiogram should be performed to assess the valve repair and quantify any residual regurgitation. Left ventricular dimensions would be expected to return to normal within a few months of surgery. Anticoagulation with warfarin is used by many surgeons for 3 months after surgery, especially if there has been postoperative atrial fibrillation. Long-term low-dose aspirin is usually recommended for 3 months, and annual or 2-yearly echocardiography.

AORTIC REGURGITATION

This valve abnormality may occur in isolation, in combination with AS or in patients with rheumatic heart disease and with mitral valve disease.

The incompetent aortic valve allows regurgitation of blood from the aorta to the left ventricle during diastole for as long as the aortic diastolic pressure exceeds the left ventricular diastolic pressure. The most common cause in developed countries is degenerative valve disease. Two-thirds of cases are a result of degeneration of a trileaflet or bicuspid valve.

CASE 4 SCENARIO: MR AL WITH MILD EXERTIONAL DYSPNOEA

Mr AL, a 56-year-old man, presents with mild exertional dyspnoea. He thinks he may have had a heart murmur noticed over 5 years ago but this was not investigated at the time.

Symptoms and Signs
What questions would you ask Mr AL?
'Do you think your shortness of breath is getting worse?
'I think so but I am getting older and have put on some weight this year.'
'Have you been short of breath at night and had to sleep sitting up on pillows? (orthopnoea)
'Have you ever woken at night gasping for breath? (PND)
'No.'
'Have you had high blood pressure?'
'Yes.'
'Have you been treated for that?'
'Yes I take amlodipine tablets – 10 mg I think.'
'Has the blood pressure been under good control?'
'My doctor always seems happy with it.'
'Do you know your cholesterol level?'
'About 5, I think.'
'Is there a history of heart disease in the family?'
'My father had a heart attack when he was about 80.'
'Have you had any other problems with your health – kidney trouble, liver trouble, a stroke?'
'No.'
'Are you a smoker?'
'I stopped 15 years ago but did smoke 2 packets a day for over 20 years.'
'Have you had problems with arthritis or rashes (seronegative arthropathies)?'
'Have you had psoriasis?'
'Have you had pain and stiffness in your back?'
'Has this been investigated?'
'What were you told was the diagnosis?'
'Was any treatment recommended?'

As with other valve problems, dyspnoea is the main symptom but rarely develops before the regurgitation is severe and the left ventricle considerably dilated.

What examination would you perform?
Of course a complete cardiovascular examination is indicated.

- **General signs:** Marfan syndrome, ankylosing spondylitis or one of the other seronegative arthropathies – these are all associated with aortic regurgitation (AR).
- **Pulse and blood pressure:** the pulse is characteristically collapsing, a 'water hammer'[1] pulse; there may be a wide pulse pressure. This sign is most obvious if the clinician raises the patient's arm while feeling the radial pulse with the lifting hand. A *bisferiens* pulse (from the Latin 'to beat twice') may be a sign of severe AR or of combined AR and AS. It is best assessed at the carotid artery, where two beats can be felt in each cardiac cycle. It is probably caused by a Venturi effect in the aorta related to rapid ejection of blood and brief in-drawing of the aortic wall, leading to a diminution of the pulse followed by a rebound increase. It was a particular favourite of Galen's.
- **Neck:** prominent carotid pulsations (Corrigan's sign).
- **Palpation:** when the regurgitation is severe the apex beat is characteristically displaced and hyperkinetic. If the regurgitation is very severe a diastolic thrill may be felt at the left sternal edge when the patient sits up and breathes out.
- **Auscultation:** A2 (the aortic component of the second heart sound) may be soft; there is a decrescendo high-pitched diastolic murmur beginning immediately after the second heart sound and extending for a variable time into diastole – it is loudest at the third and fourth left intercostal spaces; a systolic ejection murmur is usually present (due to associated AS or to torrential flow across an aortic valve of normal diameter).

  An *Austin Flint murmur* may be present. This is a low-pitched rumbling mid-diastolic and presystolic murmur audible at the apex (the regurgitant jet from the aortic valve causes the anterior mitral valve leaflet to shudder). It can be distinguished from mitral stenosis because S1 (the first heart sound) is not loud and there is no opening snap.
- **Signs indicating severe chronic AR:**
  - collapsing pulse; wide pulse pressure (systolic pressure 80 mmHg more than the diastolic)
  - long decrescendo diastolic murmur
  - left ventricular S3 (third heart sound)
  - soft A2
  - Austin Flint murmur
  - signs of left ventricular failure.
- **Causes of AR:** the disease may affect the valve alone or involve the aortic root, and may be acute or chronic. Patients with a bicuspid valve more often have aortic root involvement – dilation – and can be at risk of aortic dissection

- Causes of chronic AR:
  1. valvular – rheumatic (rarely the only murmur in this case); congenital (e.g. bicuspid valve; ventricular septal defect – an associated prolapse of the aortic cusp is not uncommon); seronegative arthropathy, especially ankylosing spondylitis
  2. aortic root dilation (murmur may be maximal at the right sternal border) – Marfan syndrome; aortitis (e.g. seronegative arthropathies, rheumatoid arthritis, tertiary syphilis); dissecting aneurysm.

The examination reveals:
- A blood pressure of 140/60
- No dyspnoea at rest
- A collapsing pulse
- Corrigan's sign
- A displaced apex beat
- No S3

- A long early diastolic murmur maximal at the base of the heart and with the patient leaning forward and in deep expiration.
- A 2/6 systolic ejection murmur in the aortic area, just audible into the neck
- No thrill.

Investigations
What would be your next step?
An echocardiogram is clearly necessary at this stage.

What information might that provide?
The transthoracic (Fig. 2.4) or transoesophageal echocardiography can give information about:
1. the valve anatomy – trileaflet or bicuspid
2. the direction of the regurgitant jet – central or eccentric

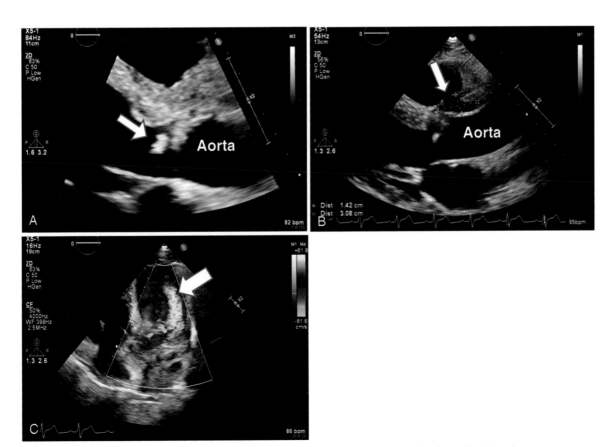

FIG. 2.4 **(A)** Infective endocarditis (IE) of the aortic valve with large vegetation (arrow) and an abscess **(B)**. **(C)** Severe aortic regurgitation jet due to IE in the same patient.

3. the likely mechanism of the regurgitation – aortic root dilation causing normal cusps to fail to coapt (central jet), or prolapse or retraction of a cusp (eccentric jet)
4. assessment of the severity of the AR (see Box 2.2)
5. measurement of LV dimensions and function – these should be indexed for body surface area (BSA) for small patients (BSA <1.6 m^2)
6. 3D echo and strain rate imaging and tissue Doppler measurements may be helpful when LV function is borderline

Measurement of the dimensions of the aortic root and ascending aorta should be made in four places:
1. the annulus
2. the sinuses of Valsalva
3. the sinotubular (aortotubular) junction
4. the tubular ascending aorta.

There are three variations in the anatomy:
1. aortic root aneurysms (sinuses of Valsalva >45 mm)
2. tubular ascending aortic aneurysm (sinuses of Valsalva <40–45 mm)
3. isolated AR (all diameters <40 mm).

These measurements should also be adjusted for BSA for large and small people.

If the echo measurements are equivocal cardiac magnetic resonance scanning can be used to measure the regurgitant fraction.

CT can be used to measure the aortic root dimensions when there is doubt and will more accurately define the anatomy of the ascending aorta and arch.

The echocardiogram shows:
- a bicuspid aortic valve
- no significant valve gradient
- a large regurgitant jet into the left ventricle
- dilation of the aortic root with a maximum diameter of 50 mm at the sinotubular junction
- left ventricular end-diastolic dimension of 72 mm
- left ventricular end-systolic dimension of 52 mm
- an ejection fraction of approximately 55%.

The CT scan shows a partly calcified aortic valve. The aortic root maximum dimension is 50 mm with no dilation of the ascending or transverse aortas.[7]

Surgery in Severe Aortic Regurgitation
What would you recommend to the patient?
There is a clear indication here for surgery (Box 2.2).

Aortic enlargement without severe AR
These patients may need surgery to protect them from aortic dissection. The risk of dissection depends on the cause of the abnormality and the size of the root.

> **BOX 2.2**
> **AR Management**
>
> 1. Significant aortic enlargement – surgery
> 2. Aortic root dimensions not significantly increased, but symptoms and severe AR present – surgery
> 3. Severe AR without symptoms but:
>   - LVEF <50% or
>   - LVEDD >70 mm or
>   - LVESD >50 mm (>25 mm/m^2 BSA)
>   – surgery
> 4. Severe AR without symptoms but:
>   - LVEF >50% and
>   - LVEDD <70 mm and
>   - LVESD <50 mm (<25 mm/m^2 BSA)
>   – regular review but consider surgery if LV dimensions rapidly increase.

AR=aortic regurgitation; BSA=body surface area; LVEDD=left ventricular end-diastolic diameter; LVEF=left ventricular ejection fraction; LVESD=left ventricular end-systolic diameter.

- Bicuspid valve – consider surgery when root size >55 mm, or >50 mm if other risk factors are present:
  - coarctation,
  - family history of aortic dissection,
  - hypertension, rapid increase in size (>3 mm/year),
  - planning pregnancy.
- Marfan syndrome – when root size >45 mm, or >40 mm if there are extra-aortic features of Marfan.
- Need for other valve surgery or coronary artery bypass graft (CABG) – when root size >45 mm.
- Native valve resuspension in the repaired aortic root is desirable if the valve is morphologically normal.

Mr AL asks if he can have a transarterial valve implantation (TAVI).

- TAVI is generally not indicated for the treatment of AR because of the increased risk of paravalvular leak. It is certainly contraindicated when there is a need for aortic root repair.

Cardiac catheterisation shows no obstructive coronary disease. Aortic root replacement and valve replacement with a mechanical prosthesis is performed. He has requested a mechanical valve because of his reluctance to consider the possibility of further surgery in the future. He is aware of the need for anticoagulation with warfarin.

Long-Term Management and Follow-Up
Mr AL has an uncomplicated stay in hospital and goes home after 7 days.

What should his target INR be?

Modern bileaflet mechanical valves have a low or medium thrombogenicity (unlike older tilting-disc or ball-in-cage valves). For patients without other risk factors for thrombosis:

- atrial fibrillation
- mitral stenosis
- previous thromboembolism
- left ventricular ejection fraction (LVEF) <35%

an INR of 2.5–3.0 is recommended.

The valve company has given him a home INR testing machine. He asks if you advise him to use this or go to his local doctor where there is an INR clinic.

There is now evidence that, for sensible patients, home INR testing reduces the variability in INR results and the frequency of adverse clinical events.

He should be encouraged to measure his own INRs but to have testing done at his doctor's surgery until he has experience in how to perform the test and in making adjustments to his warfarin dosage. He must have someone he can contact if concerned about his INR reading and an action plan for the management of serious bleeding (e.g. haematuria, haematemesis).

He asks if he should take or avoid aspirin when taking warfarin.

Antiplatelet drugs are generally to be avoided for anticoagulated patients. Exceptions include those with severe atherosclerotic disease and a low bleeding risk and patients having angioplasty and stent insertion (see Chapter 3).

What follow-up should be arranged?

Regular echocardiography is indicated to help assess:

- LV function and dimensions, which should return to normal over the first few months
- the presence of a paravalvular leak; small leaks are common and rarely cause trouble, whereas large ones can result in significant AR and valve haemolysis
- the size of the repaired aortic root
- the gradient across the valve; the peak gradient is usually 25 mmHg or less but use of a prosthesis which is too small my result in a significant gradient.

The patient's INR measurements should be reviewed regularly and he should keep a record of his results and the dates of the tests.

What should he do if he needs non-cardiac surgery?

- For minor surgery and if the surgeon thinks it safe from the point of view of risk of haemorrhage, it may be reasonable to allow the INR to fall to 2.0 for the perioperative period. Otherwise warfarin must be stopped 4–5 days before surgery and subcutaneous enoxaparin given in therapeutic doses (1 mg/kg twice daily) until 12 hours before surgery. It should be continued in the postoperative period until warfarin has been restarted and the INR reaches 2.0.
- Patients with valve replacements require antibiotic prophylaxis for dental and surgical procedures.

Mr AL has been to a cardiac rehabilitation course and now feels confident to go back to work and resume normal physical activity. He feels his exercise tolerance is back to normal. He has had no problems with his sternal wound.

He and his wife are both able to hear his mechanical valve sounds but have not found this disturbing.

He feels increasingly confident about his home INR monitoring and is looking forward to a 6-week overseas holiday later in the year. He expects to be able to manage his warfarin himself while he is away.

REFERENCES

1. Baumgartner H, Falk V, Bax J, De Bonis M, Hamm C, Holm P, et al. 2017 ESC/EACTS guidelines for the management of valvular heart disease. *Eur Heart J* 2017;**38**(36):2739–86.
2. Thourani VH, Suri RM, Gunter RL, Sheng S, O'Brien SM, Ailawadi G, et al. Contemporary real-world outcomes of surgical aortic valve replacement in 141,905 low-risk, intermediate-risk and high-risk patients. *Ann Thorac Surg* 2015;**99**(1):55–61.
3. Heneghan C, Ward A, Perera R, Self-Monitoring Trialist Collaboration, Bankhead C, Fuller A, et al. Self-monitoring of oral anti-coagulation: systematic review and meta-analysis of individual patient data. *Lancet* 2012;**379**(9813):322–34.
4. Eikelboom JW, Connolly SJ, Brueckmann M, Granger CB, Kappetein AP, Mack MJ, et al. RE_ALIGN investigators. Dabigatran versus warfarin in patients with mechanical heart valves. *N Engl J Med* 2013;**369**(13):1206–14.
5. Le Tourneau T, Richardson M, Juthier F, Modine T, Fayad G, Polge AS, et al. Echocardiography predictors and prognostic value of pulmonary artery systolic pressure in chronic organic mitral regurgitation. *Heart* 2010;**96**(16):1311–17.
6. Enriquez-Sarano M, Tajik AJ, Schaff HV, Orszulak TA, Bailey KR, Frye RL, et al. Echocardiographic prediction of survival after surgical correction of organic mitral regurgitation. *Circulation* 1994;**90**(2):830–7.
7. Klodas E, Enriquez-Sarano M, Tajik AJ, Mullany CJ, Bailey KR, Seward JB, et al. Optimising timing of surgical correction in patients with severe aortic regurgitation: role of symptoms. *J Am Coll Cardiol* 1997;**30**(3):746–52.

ST Elevation Myocardial Infarction

CASE 5 SCENARIO: JOHN WITH CHEST PAIN

A 60-year-old man named John with a history of diabetes and hypertension presents to the hospital emergency room with severe retrosternal chest pain. The pain started 2 hours previously and continued despite his self-medicating with antacids. He smokes 20 cigarettes a day. He is sweating and looks pale. The examination is unremarkable except for a blood pressure of 154/92 mmHg. His usual medications include: metformin 1000 mg twice daily and perindopril 2.5 mg daily. He also uses fluticasone puffer for his asthma.

What is the most appropriate next step in management?

1. *Arrange blood test including troponin (cTnI) and wait for the result. Call the cardiologist if the result is abnormal.*
2. *Perform immediate ECG and consider reperfusion strategy if indicated.*
3. *Insert an intravenous line and order a chest x-ray.*
4. *Arrange bedside echocardiography to assess for regional wall motion abnormalities and right ventricular size.*

John had an ECG showing ST elevation in LII, LIII and aVF (double arrow) with reciprocal ST depression (single arrow) in LI and aVL (Fig. 3.1).

John has a number of risk factors for coronary artery disease (CAD) including his age, male sex, diabetes, hypertension and current smoker. John is also presenting with typical symptoms of myocardial infarction.

COMMON SYMPTOMS OF ISCHAEMIA

These include:
- deep, poorly localised chest pain, pressure, tightness or heaviness
- pain radiating to the neck, jaw, shoulders, back or arms
- indigestion or heartburn, nausea or vomiting
- diaphoresis
- dyspnoea
- weakness, dizziness, lightheadedness or loss of consciousness
- characteristic pain is less common in the elderly and in women
- atypical presentations are also common in diabetic patients.

ROLE OF INITIAL ECG AND SERIAL TROPONIN IN ACUTE MYOCARDIAL INFARCTION
ECG[1]

- It is recommended that a patient with acute chest pain or other symptoms suggestive of a myocardial infarction (MI) receive a 12-lead ECG within 10 minutes

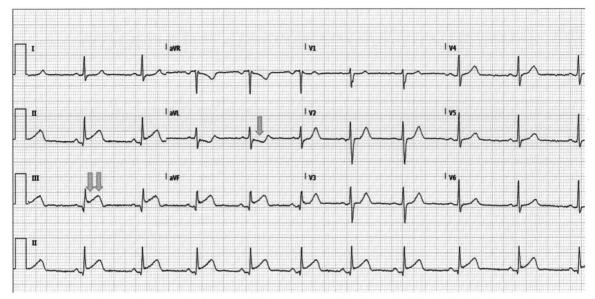

FIG. 3.1 Echocardiogram showing acute inferior myocardial infarction with ST elevation (double arrow) in LII, LIII and aVF and reciprocal ST depression (single arrow) in LI and aVL.

of the first medical contact. This initial assessment is to rapidly identify patients with an acute ST-segment elevation MI (STEMI) for consideration of emergency reperfusion therapy if clinically indicated. Restoring coronary patency as promptly as possible is a key determinant of short-term and long-term outcomes.

- A normal ECG does not rule out MI. ECG in the setting of non-ST elevation MI (NSTEMI) may be normal in more than one-third of patients. However, the ECG is the sole test required for selecting patients for emergency reperfusion either with fibrinolytic therapy or by primary angioplasty. Patients with STEMI who present within 12 hours of the onset of chest pain / discomfort should have a reperfusion strategy implemented promptly. Ongoing symptoms require frequent follow-up 12-lead ECGs (15 minutes apart) to rapidly detect ST-segment elevation and diagnose eligibility for a reperfusion strategy.

Troponin[2–4]

Troponin is a highly sensitive biomarker of myocardial injury that is used in the diagnosis of acute MI and for risk stratification of patients with acute coronary symptoms. Troponin levels become elevated in the bloodstream within 1–3 hours after MI and should be measured at hospital presentation.

Though new criteria acknowledge that elevations in biomarkers are fundamental to the diagnosis of acute MI, when appropriate ECG changes are present (ST elevation) waiting for cTnI results may cause unacceptable delay in reperfusion.

ADDITIONAL INVESTIGATIONS INCLUDING CXR AND ECHOCARDIOGRAPHY

Additional investigations including chest x-ray (CXR) and echocardiography may be useful in selective cases, but in this case it may cause unnecessary delay in reperfusion.

A CXR is useful for assessing heart size, evidence of heart failure and other abnormalities including a widened mediastinum (aortic dissection), but should not delay reperfusion treatment when that is indicated. In selected cases, when clinically indicated, CT pulmonary angiogram may be used to exclude pulmonary embolism or a CT aortogram to exclude aortic dissection may be considered. Delay in the diagnosis of MI can cause the window of opportunity for immediate thrombolysis or primary angioplasty to be missed.

Bedside echocardiography can be quite useful in specific patients when the diagnosis is in doubt. It may show segmental left ventricular dysfunction in the distribution of the infarct-related artery. It may also be useful in excluding other serious causes of chest pain. It may show a dilated aorta (raising the possibility of dissection), acute aortic regurgitation, pericardial effusion, a dissection flap in the case of aortic dissection or a dilated right ventricle in the case of a large pulmonary embolism.

You discussed John's management with the nearest cardiologist in a tertiary hospital, where his ECG was faxed. John was diagnosed with acute inferior MI.

MANAGEMENT STRATEGIES OF ACUTE MYOCARDIAL INFARCTION

Important management strategies for John include:
- aspirin, P2Y12 inhibitors (clopidogrel, ticagrelor, prasugrel) and other antiplatelet agents, heparin and intravenous fentanyl
- immediate thrombolysis and transfer for coronary angiography
- immediate transfer to a tertiary hospital with cardiac catheterisation facility for consideration of primary percutaneous transluminal coronary angioplasty (PTCA)
- ECG monitorng and access to a defibrillator.

Acute Management[1]
- The most important initial requirement is access to a defibrillator to avoid early cardiac death from reversible arrhythmias. It has also been reported that conscious STEMI patients resuscitated from cardiac arrest and treated with PTCA can be expected to have the same prognosis as those treated with PTCA who have not suffered a cardiac arrest.

Common Antiplatelet Drugs
Aspirin
- Aspirin (ASA) 300 mg orally as soon as the diagnosis is made, followed by 100 mg daily.
- ASA inhibits thromboxane A_2 synthesis by irreversibly acetylating cyclooxygenase-1 in platelets and megakaryocytes.
- Platelets are unable to regenerate cyclooxygenase; the immediate antithrombotic effect of ASA remains for the lifespan of the platelet (8–10 days).
- In the ISIS-2 (Second International Study of Infarct Survival) trial, patients were randomly allocated to treatment with aspirin, streptokinase, both or placebo within the first 24 hours of suspected or evolving MI. The 5-week cardiovascular mortality was reduced by 23% during ASA treatment, from 11.8% to 9.4%.[5]

P2Y12 inhibition (Table 3.1)
- It is recommended that patients be given ticagrelor 180 mg loading followed by 90 mg twice daily, or prasugrel 60 mg orally, then 10 mg daily or clopidogrel 300–600 mg orally and then 75 mg daily.
- The new-generation P2Y12 inhibitors (ticagrelor or prasugrel) are preferred to clopidogrel owing to their superior efficacy and they should be considered as soon as the diagnosis is made and, unless contraindicated, should be continued (in addition to aspirin) for 12 months following ACS.
- If the patient is likely to have significant triple-vessel disease or left main artery disease (based on ECG findings and clinically), use of P2Y12 inhibitors (clopidogrel, ticagrelor or prasugrel) should be delayed until angiography is done and the coronary anatomy is known. In this situation, use of these agents could delay urgent bypass surgery and increase the risk of serious bleeding.
- Clopidogrel is recommended for patients with fibrinolysis who cannot receive ticagrelor or prasugrel, as an adjunctive agent, or for those requiring additional oral anticoagulation (triple therapy) for another indication (e.g. metallic valve or atrial fibrillation).

Heparin
- Low-molecular-weight heparin (enoxaparin), 1 mg/kg subcutaneous BD (unless there is renal impairment), or unfractionated heparin, 60–70 units/kg IV and infusion 12–15 units/kg per hour with target aPTT (activated partial thromboplastin time) 1.5–2.5 times control is recommended in intermediate- to high-risk patients with acute coronary syndromes.
- Unfractionated heparin is often preferred if patients are to go to the catheterisation lab, where the ACT (activated clotting time) can be measured and dosage adjusted to achieve a predictable level of anticoagulation.

Glycoprotein IIb/IIIa inhibitors
- Trials of GPIIb/IIIa inhibitors (abciximab, tirofiban, eptifibatide) in combination with heparin among acute coronary syndrome patients were conducted in an era prior to the routine use of P2Y12 inhibitors.
- They are recommended in specific high-risk patients and in patients who have a large thrombus load detected during angiography.
- O_2 supplementation should be considered only if the patient is hypoxic (S_aO_2 <93%) and has no history of chronic lung disease with CO_2 retention.
- In the presence of ongoing chest pain, sublingual nitroglycerin (1 spray or glyceryl trinitrate (GTN) tablet 0.3–0.6 mg at onset of attack) should be given every 5 minutes for up to three dosages (unless the patient is hypotensive).
- IV morphine (2.5–15 mg diluted in 4–5 mL water for injection, slow IV) or fentanyl (25–100 µg IV) can also be considered for ongoing chest pain.

TABLE 3.1
Common Antiplatelet Drugs

Drugs	Dosage	Mechanism	Important Side Effects	Note
Aspirin	300 mg orally initially, followed by 100 mg daily.	Inhibits thromboxane A_2 synthesis by irreversibly acetylating cyclooxygenase.	Can cause non-fatal extracranial haemorrhage in 1–2 per 1000 patients treated per year. Increased risk of intracranial haemorrhage in about 1 per 1000 patients treated for 3 years.	Unless contraindicated, should be continued long term following ACS. Aspirin reduces the risk of serious vascular events in patients at high risk by about 23%. Recommended as the 1st-line antiplatelet drug.
Ticagrelor	180 mg orally, followed by 90 mg twice daily.	Ticagrelor is a potent, reversibly binding, direct-acting P2Y12 receptor blocker.	Bleeding. Dyspnoea in 14% of patients. Bradyarrhythmias including AV block.	Should not be used in presence of atrioventricular conduction defect, asthma/COPD, previous intracranial bleed.
Prasugrel	60 mg orally followed by 10 mg daily.	Prasugrel is a 3rd-generation thienopyridine, an ADP receptor antagonist that is a potent inhibitor of platelet activation and aggregation.	Life-threatening and fatal bleeding. Contraindicated in patients with active bleeding, severe hepatic impairment.	Considered in a patient who is planned to have PTCA. Should not be used in patients >75 years, body weight <60 kg, H/O TIA/stroke.
Clopidogrel	300–600 mg orally followed by 75 mg daily.	Metabolised in the liver to active compounds that bind to the ADP receptors on platelets.	Compared with aspirin, clopidogrel is associated with lower risk of GI haemorrhage, increased risk of diarrhoea and skin rash. Severe neutropenia has been noted in 0.1% of patients.	Contraindicated in severe liver disease, pregnancy and lactation.

ACS=acute coronary syndrome; AV=atrioventricular; COPD=chronic obstructive pulmonary disease; TIA=transient ischaemic attack.

Reperfusion: Primary Angioplasty (PTCA) vs Thrombolysis

Angioplasty

Primary PTCA is the preferred reperfusion therapy in patients with STEMI, provided it can be performed within 90 minutes of first medical contact by appropriately qualified interventional cardiologists in a suitable facility. Otherwise, fibrinolytic therapy is preferred for those without contraindications.

Meta-analysis[6] of 23 randomised trials (total 7739 patients) of primary angioplasty (PTCA) versus intravenous thrombolytic therapy for acute MI shows PTCA to be superior to fibrinolytic therapy in reducing mortality, recurrent MI and stroke. Compared with fibrinolysis, primary PCI provides an additional benefit of 1.5–2 lives saved per 100 patients treated.

A total of eight studies (1837 patients) have used streptokinase and an additional 15 studies have used tPA (5902 patients). Overall, the patients assigned to

PTCA were less likely to die (odds ratio (OR) 0.73; 95% confidence interval (CI): 0.62, 0.86), have a non-fatal infarction (OR 0.35; 95% CI: 0.27, 0.45), have a haemorrhagic stroke (OR 0.05; 95% CI: 0.006, 0.35) or experience the combined end point of death, re-infarction or stroke (OR 0.53; 95% CI: 0.45, 0.63), than those assigned to thrombolysis. This was true for both short- and long-term outcomes.

Fibrinolysis should be considered early on if PTCA is not readily available, particularly in rural and remote areas or when there is an unacceptable delay (more than 90 minutes after first medical contact) in transferring the patient to an angioplasty facility. Compared with control groups, fibrinolysis reduces overall mortality at 35 days with a relative risk of 0.82 (95% CI: 0.77, 0.87) based on data from nine trials involving 58,600 patients. This benefit was greater among those patients with anterior MI. The impact on mortality through myocardial salvage is greatest in the first hour after symptom onset and diminishes with time.[7]

Reperfusion is not routinely recommended in patients who present more than 12 hours after symptom onset who are asymptomatic and haemodynamically stable.

Thrombolysis[1,8]
- There are four fibrinolytic agents currently available in Australia: streptokinase and the tissue fibrin-specific fibrinolytic agents alteplase, reteplase and tenecteplase.

- Fibrin-specific fibrinolytic agents have been shown to reduce mortality compared with streptokinase in patients with STEMI.
- Streptokinase may be associated with a lower incidence of intracranial haemorrhage, particularly in older people.
- There is evidence that streptokinase may be less effective in Aboriginal and Torres Strait Islander peoples because of their high incidence of streptococcal infection (and thus streptococcal antibodies). Streptokinase is an inappropriate choice for Aboriginal and Torres Strait Islander patients or patients with previous exposure to the drug.

The treatment options of immediate thrombolysis vs transfer for percutaneous angioplasty were discussed with John's cardiologist, who prescribed aspirin 300 mg, ticagrelor 180 mg and heparin 5000 units.

However, while you were on the phone John suddenly developed ventricular fibrillation. As he was on an ECG monitor, the arrhythmia was recognised immediately and he was successfully reverted to sinus rhythm by a single shock with a defibrillator, without the need for cardiopulmonary resuscitation. He was transferred to the nearest tertiary hospital for primary angioplasty within 30 minutes. He was immediately taken to the cardiac catheterisation laboratory (bypassing the emergency department) and had a stent inserted into his totally occluded right coronary artery, with establishment of TIMI III flow (Fig. 3.2).

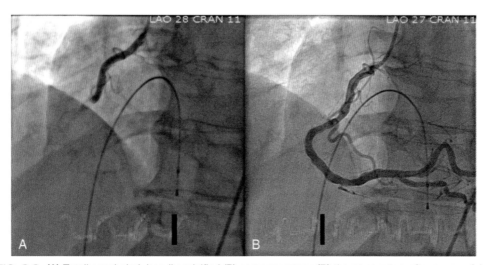

FIG. 3.2 **(A)** Totally occluded, heavily calcified (R) coronary artery; **(B)** the same artery after successful stenting. STEMI generally results from occlusive thrombus. Restoring coronary patency as promptly as possible by primary angioplasty or fibrinolytic therapy is a key determinant of short-term and long-term outcome.

QUESTIONS

1. What is the incidence of MI in Australia?
2. How do you define MI?
3. What is the pathogenesis of MI?
4. Classify the types of MI.
5. What ECG changes are present in a STEMI?

MYOCARDIAL INFARCTION IN AUSTRALIA

Acute MI remains the leading cause of death in Australia and worldwide. It is estimated that over 350,000 Australians have had a heart attack at some time in their lives. Each year, around 54,000 Australians have a heart attack. This equates to one heart attack every nine minutes. On average, cardiovascular disease accounted for nearly 30% of all deaths in Australia in 2014.[9]

DEFINITIONS OF MYOCARDIAL INFARCTION

Acute MI refers to cardiomyocyte necrosis in a clinical setting consistent with acute myocardial ischaemia. Recent definitions of MI are based heavily on the presence of cardiac biomarkers (troponins). A combination of criteria must be met for the diagnosis of acute MI.[4]

Definitions of myocardial infarction include:

- Detection of an increase and then decrease in a cardiac biomarker, preferably high-sensitivity cardiac troponin, with at least one value above the 99th percentile of the upper reference limit plus at least one of the following:
  - symptoms of ischaemia
  - new, or presumed new, significant ST-segment–T wave (ST–T) changes or new left bundle branch block
  - development of pathological Q waves on an ECG
  - imaging evidence of a new loss of viable myocardium or new regional wall motion abnormality
  - intracoronary thrombus detected on angiography or autopsy.[4]

PATHOGENESIS OF MYOCARDIAL INFARCTION

- Atherosclerosis is a continuing process affecting mainly large- and medium-sized arteries. It can begin in childhood and progress throughout a person's lifetime.
- Unstable atherosclerotic plaques may rupture, leading to the formation of a platelet-rich thrombus that partially or completely occludes the artery and causes acute ischaemic symptoms.

CLINICAL CLASSIFICATION OF MYOCARDIAL INFARCTION

The term 'acute coronary syndrome' (ACS) refers to a spectrum of conditions compatible with acute myocardial ischaemia or infarction that are usually caused by an abrupt reduction in coronary blood flow.

These conditions include unstable angina, STEMI and NSTEMI. The presentation of unstable angina includes angina at rest, new-onset severe angina, and angina increasing in intensity, duration and/or frequency.

There are many different ways to classify acute MIs. A common clinical classification system based on ECG findings distinguishes two MI types:

- STEMI – which is marked by persistent (over 20 minutes) ST elevation or new left bundle branch block.
- NSTEMI – there is no persistent ST elevation or new left bundle branch block; ECG changes may include transient ST-segment elevation, ST-segment depression or T-wave changes, or the ECG may be normal.[10-13]

STEMI generally results from a red, fibrin-rich, occlusive thrombus (see Fig. 3.2). Restoring coronary patency as promptly as possible by primary angioplasty or fibrinolytic therapy is a key determinant of short-term and long-term outcome. In patients with STEMI, 'time equals muscle', and a delay in treatment can often lead to irreversible muscle damage (Fig. 3.3), heart failure, death and other complications that adversely affect prognosis and quality of life.

In contrast, NSTEMI is generally associated with a white, platelet-rich, partially occlusive thrombus. The clinical spectrum of NSTEMI varies, and the treatment strategy, including the timing of coronary angiography or revascularisation, depends on risk assessment using common clinical risk assessment scores (discussed in Chapter 4).[11-13]

Unstable angina is defined as myocardial ischaemia at rest or on minimal exertion in the absence of cardiomyocyte necrosis. Patients with unstable angina have a better prognosis than do those with NSTEMI and are less likely to benefit from early invasive angiography or revascularisation.

In addition to these categories, MI is classified into various types, based on pathological, clinical and prognostic differences, along with different treatment strategies (Box 3.1).[14]

BOX 3.1
Universal Definitions of Myocardial Injury and Myocardial Infarction

CRITERIA FOR MYOCARDIAL INJURY

The term myocardial injury should be used when there is evidence of elevated cardiac troponin values (cTn) with at least one value above the 99th percentile upper reference limit (URL). The myocardial injury is considered acute if there is a rise and/or fall of cTn values.

CRITERIA FOR ACUTE MYOCARDIAL INFARCTION (TYPES 1, 2 AND 3 MI)

The term acute myocardial infarction should be used when there is acute myocardial injury with clinical evidence of acute myocardial ischaemia and with detection of a rise and/or fall of cTn values with at least one value above the 99th percentile URL and at least one of the following:

- Symptoms of myocardial ischaemia;
- New ischaemic ECG changes;
- Development of pathological Q waves;
- Imaging evidence of new loss of viable myocardium or new regional wall motion abnormality in a pattern consistent with an ischaemic aetiology;
- Identification of a coronary thrombus by angiography or autopsy (not for type 2 or 3 MIs).

Post-mortem demonstration of acute atherothrombosis in the artery supplying the infarcted myocardium meets criteria for type 1 MI.

Evidence of an imbalance between myocardial oxygen supply and demand unrelated to acute atherothrombosis meets criteria for type 2 MI.

Cardiac death in patients with symptoms suggestive of myocardial ischaemia and presumed new ischaemic ECG changes before cTn values become available or abnormal meets criteria for type 3 MI.

CRITERIA FOR CORONARY PROCEDURE-RELATED MYOCARDIAL INFARCTION (TYPES 4 AND 5 MI)

Percutaneous coronary intervention (PCI)-related MI is termed type 4a MI.

Coronary artery bypass grafting (CABG)-related MI is termed type 5 MI.

Coronary procedure-related MI ≤48 hours after the index procedure is arbitrarily defined by an elevation of cTn values >5 times for type 4a MI and >10 times for type 5 MI of the 99th percentile URL in patients with normal baseline values. In addition with at least one of the following:

- New ischaemic ECG changes (this criterion is related to type 4a MI only);
- Development of new pathological Q waves;
- Imaging evidence of loss of viable myocardium that is presumed to be new and in a pattern consistent with an ischaemic aetiology;
- Angiographic findings consistent with a procedural flow-limiting complication such as coronary dissection, occlusion of a major epicardial artery or graft, side-branch occlusion-thrombus, disruption of collateral flow or distal embolisation.

Isolated development of new pathological Q waves meets the type 4a MI or type 5 MI criteria with either revascularisation procedure if cTn values are elevated and rising but less than the prespecified thresholds for PCI and CABG.

Other types of 4 MI include type 4b MI stent thrombosis and type 4c MI restenosis that both meet type 1 MI criteria.

Post-mortem demonstration of a procedure-related thrombus meets the type 4a MI criteria or type 4b MI criteria if associated with a stent.

CRITERIA FOR PRIOR OR SILENT/ UNRECOGNISED MYOCARDIAL INFARCTION

Any one of the following criteria meets the diagnosis for prior or silent/unrecognised MI:

- Abnormal Q waves with or without symptoms in the absence of non-ischaemic causes;
- Imaging evidence of loss of viable myocardium in a pattern consistent with ischaemic aetiology;
- Pathoanatomical findings of a prior MI.

CABG=coronary artery bypass grafting; cTn=cardiac troponin; ECG=electrocardiogram; MI=myocardial infarction; PCI=percutaneous coronary intervention; URL=upper reference limit.
(From Thygesen K, Alpert JS, Jaffe AS, Chaitman BR, Bax JJ, Morrow DA, et al.; The Executive Group on behalf of the Joint European Society of Cardiology (ESC)/American College of Cardiology (ACC)/American Heart Association (AHA)/World Heart Federation (WHF) Task Force for the Universal Definition of Myocardial Infarction. Fourth universal definition of myocardial infarction. *J Am Coll Cardiol* 2018;72(18):2235, with permission.)

ECG Diagnostic Criteria of ST Elevation Myocardial Infarction[1,10,15,16]

ST elevation in acute MI is typically confined to a single vascular territory and is convex upward. Often there is reciprocal ST depression in the opposite leads. In the early stages of acute MI, the ECG may show tall, peaked T waves followed by ST-segment elevation (Table 3.2).

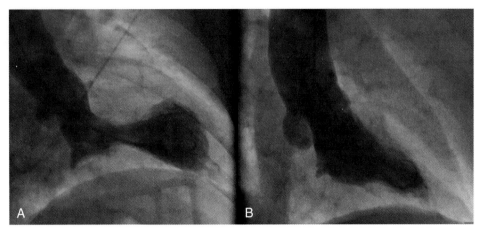

FIG. 3.3 Ventriculography: **(A)** significant mid-distal anterior to apical akinesia following large anterior STEMI; **(B)** normal left ventricular systolic function.

TABLE 3.2
Localisation of Infarct Artery Involved and ECG Findings in Patients With Acute Myocardial Infarction[10,11]

Location	Artery Involved	ECG Features
Inferior	Right coronary artery (RCA)	Greater ST elevation in LIII compared with LII ST depression in LI and aVL
	Left circumflex (L Cx)	Isoelectric or elevated ST segment in LI, aVL, V5 and V6 (in addition to ST elevation in LII, LIII and aVF)
Right ventricle infarction	Proximal RCA	ST elevation in V4R (right-sided chest lead) ST elevation in V1 associated with ST elevation in II, III and aVF
Posterior	Posterior descending artery – usually a branch of the RCA	ECG changes are mirror image of an anteroseptal MI: • R/S ratio in V1 or V2 >1 • Hyperacute ST–T-wave changes: i.e. ST depression and large, inverted T waves in V1 to V3 Posterior infarction is confirmed by the presence of ST elevation and Q waves in the posterior leads (V7 to V9)
Anterior	Left anterior descending artery (LAD)	Anterior=V2 to V5 Anteroseptal=V1 to V3 Extensive anterior=V1 to V6, I and aVL
	Proximal LAD	Prominent ST elevation in I and aVL and inferior ST depression is consistent with proximal LAD occlusion
	Distal LAD	ST depression in aVL particularly if combined with isoelectric ST segments in the inferior leads suggests distal LAD occlusion
Lateral	• Diagonal branch of the LAD • Obtuse marginal branch of (L) Cx • Ramus intermedius (intermediate artery)	ST elevation in the lateral leads (LI, aVL, V5 and V6) Reciprocal ST depression in the inferior leads (III and aVF)

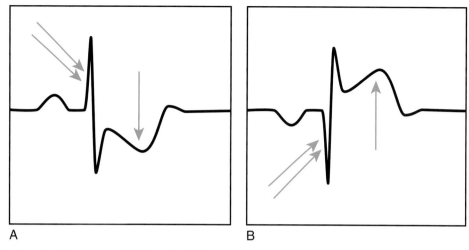

FIG. 3.4 Posterior myocardial infraction: **(A)** tall R wave (double arrow) in lead V1 with ST depression (single arrow); **(B)** (double arrow) Q wave (mirror image of large R wave from part **A**) and ST elevation (single arrow), mirror image of ST depression in part **A**.

ECG criteria for STEMI are persistent (>20 minutes) ST-segment elevation in two or more contiguous leads of:

- 2.5 mm or more ST elevation in leads V2–3 in men under 40 years, or
- 2 mm or more ST elevation in leads V2–3 in men over 40 years, or
- 1.5 mm or more ST elevation in V2–3 in women, or
- 1 mm or more ST elevation in other leads, or
- development of new left bundle branch block.

Posterior STEMI

- ECG changes (Fig. 3.4) are a mirror image of an anteroseptal MI: increased R-wave amplitude and duration (i.e. a 'pathological R wave' is a mirror image of a pathological Q)
- R/S ratio in V1 or V2 >1
- Hyperacute ST–T-wave changes: i.e. ST depression and large, upright T waves in V1–3.

A posterior MI can also be diagnosed by recording an ECG with leads V7–9 on the posterior chest wall. In practice this means running the precordial leads onto the back of the chest and placing the electrodes in the same plane as V6 (V7=left posterior axillary line, V8=tip of left scapula, V9=left paraspinal region). A posterior MI is diagnosed if there is ST elevation in any of leads V7 to V9.

John was fortunate and was discharged home on day 5 with a follow-up appointment and cardiac rehabilitation plan.

His discharge medications included aspirin 100 mg daily, ticagrelor 90 mg twice daily, atorvastatin 40 mg daily and perindopril 2.5 mg daily. His previous medications including metformin and Seretide were continued.

REFERENCES

1. Chew DP, Scott IA, Cullen L, French JK, Briffa TG, Tideman PA, et al; NHFA/CSANZ ACS Guideline 2016 Executive Working Group. National Heart Foundation of Australia and Cardiac Society of Australia and New Zealand: Australian clinical guidelines for the management of acute coronary syndromes 2016. *Heart Lung Circ* 2016;**25**:895–951.
2. Babuin L, Jaffe AS. Troponin: the biomarker of choice for the detection of cardiac injury. *CMAJ* 2005;**173**:1191–202.
3. Newby LK, Jesse RL, Babb JD, Christenson RH, De Fer TM, Diamond GA, et al. ACCF 2012 expert consensus document on practical clinical considerations in the interpretation of troponin elevations: a report of the American College of Cardiology Foundation task force on Clinical Expert Consensus Documents. *J Am Coll Cardiol* 2012;**60**: 2427–63.
4. Thygesen K, Alpert JS, Jaffe AS, Simoons ML, Chaitman BR, White HD, et al; Joint ESC/ACCF/AHA/WHF Task Force for Universal Definition of Myocardial Infarction; Authors/Task Force Members Chairpersons. Third universal definition of MI. *J Am Coll Cardiol* 2012;**60**:1581–98.
5. [No authors listed]. Randomised trial of intravenous streptokinase, oral aspirin, both or neither among 17 187 cases of suspected acute myocardial infarction: ISIS-2 (Second International Study of Infarct Survival) Collaborative Group. *Lancet* 1988;**2**:349–60.

6. Keeley EC, Boura JA, Grines CL. Primary angioplasty versus intravenous thrombolytic therapy for acute myocardial infarction: a quantitative review of 23 randomised trials. *Lancet* 2003;**361**(9351):13–20.

7. Fibrinolytic Therapy Trialists' (FTT) Collaborative Group. Indications for fibrinolytic therapy in suspected acute myocardial infarction: collaborative overview of early mortality and major morbidity results from all randomised trials of more than 1000 patients: Fibrinolytic Therapy Trialists' (FTT) Collaborative, Group. *Lancet* 1994;**343**(8893):311–22.

8. Acute Coronary Syndrome Guidelines Working Group. Guidelines for the management of acute coronary syndromes 2006. *Med J Aust* 2006;**184**(8 Suppl.):S9–29.

9. Australian Bureau of Statistics. *Causes of death, Australia,* 2013. https://www.abs.gov.au/Causes-of-Death.

10. White HD, Chew DP. Acute myocardial infarction. *Lancet* 2008;**372**(9638):570–84.

11. Amsterdam EA, Wenger NK, Brindis RG, Casey DE Jr, Ganiats TG, Holmes DR Jr, et al; ACC/AHA Task Force Members. 2014 AHA/ACC guideline for the management of patients with non-ST-elevation acute coronary syndromes: a report of the American College of Cardiology/American Heart Association Task Force on Practice Guidelines. *Circulation* 2014;**130**:e344–426.

12. Roffi M, Patrono C, Collet JP, Mueller C, Valgimigli M, Andreotti F, et al. 2015 ESC Guidelines for the management of acute coronary syndromes in patients presenting without persistent ST-segment elevation: task force for the management of acute coronary syndromes in patients presenting without persistent ST-segment elevation of the European Society of Cardiology (ESC). *Eur Heart J* 2016;**37**:267–315.

13. Task force on the management of ST-segment elevation acute myocardial infarction of the European Society of Cardiology (ESC), Steg PG, James SK, Atar D, Badano LP, Blömstrom-Lundqvist C, et al. ESC Guidelines for the management of acute myocardial infarction in patients presenting with ST-segment elevation. *Eur Heart J* 2012;**33**:2569–619.

14. Thygesen K, Alpert JS, Jaffe AS, Chaitman BR, Bax JJ, Morrow DA, et al. The Executive Group on behalf of the Joint European Society of Cardiology (ESC)/American College of Cardiology (ACC)/American Heart Association (AHA)/World Heart Federation (WHF) Task Force for the Universal Definition of Myocardial Infarction. Fourth universal definition of myocardial infarction. *J Am Coll Cardiol* 2018;**72**(18):2235.

15. Zimetbaum PJ, Josephson ME. Use of the electrocardiogram in acute myocardial infarction. *N Engl J Med* 2003;**348**:933–40.

16. Arbane M, Goy JJ. Prediction of the site of total occlusion in the left anterior descending coronary artery using admission electrocardiogram in anterior wall acute myocardial infarction. *Am J Cardiol* 2000;**85**:487–91.

CHAPTER 4

Secondary Prevention of Coronary Artery Disease

CASE 6 SCENARIO: JOHN IN CARDIAC REHAB

John is reviewed 2 weeks later in cardiac rehabilitation. He recovered well from the recent myocardial infarction. His echocardiography showed inferior hypokinesia with an ejection fraction of 45%. His total cholesterol is 7.4 mmol/L and HDL cholesterol (HDL-C) 0.8 mmol/L.

He has had no further chest pain or discomfort. He had stopped taking his atorvastatin as his friend told him the risk of serious side effects. Unfortunately, he has continued to smoke and is not very keen to continue all his medications.

Clinical questions
- *What is the role of lifestyle changes in the long-term management of John?*

- *How important are statins in secondary prevention and what are the possible side effects?*
- *What is the role and duration of dual antiplatelet drugs?*
- *What is the role of beta-blockers/ACE inhibitors in ACS?*

LIFESTYLE CHANGES IN THE LONG-TERM MANAGEMENT OF CARDIOVASCULAR DISEASE
Effect of Exercise, Smoking and Diet on Cholesterol
- Increased physical activity is related to reduced risk of cardiovascular disease and has a beneficial effect on a variety of lipid and lipoprotein variables. Despite the fact that there is a clear beneficial effect on the HDL-C concentration and improvement in triglyceride (TG) concentration, exercise training has no significant

effect on the total cholesterol or LDC-C concentrations. Low HDL-C is an important risk factor for coronary heart disease, stroke and even small increases in HDL-C may confer substantial benefit.[1]

- There is a strong and graded relation between number of pack-years smoked and risk of myocardial infarction. In a study by Moffatt, smokers had HDL-C levels 15%–20% lower than non-smokers. HDL-C levels returned to normal within 30–60 days after smoking cessation.[2] Drug therapy with bupropion or nicotine replacement is not essential and is not recommended for patients who smoke <10 cigarettes/day.

- A number of studies suggested that the Mediterranean diet can modestly lower LDL and TGs, as well as raise HDL-C.[3] Diets with low saturated fat content reduce cholesterol by 5%–10%. The traditional Mediterranean diet is characterised by a high intake of olive oil, fruit, nuts, vegetables and cereals; a moderate intake of fish and poultry; and a low intake of dairy products, red meat, processed meats and sweets (Box 4.1).

Healthy diet

- Eat at least five portions of a variety of fruit and vegetables each day. They are rich in vitamins and minerals.
- Limit the amount of saturated fat. Foods that are high in saturated fat include meat pies, sausages, butter, cream, hard cheese, cakes, biscuits and foods that contain coconut or palm oil. Eating foods that are high in unsaturated fat can help to reduce cholesterol levels. Foods high in unsaturated fat include oily fish (such as herring, mackerel, sardine, salmon), avocados, nuts and olive oil.
- Lowering salt intake can reduce the risk of a further heart attack as well as reduce the risk of other cardiovascular diseases.

In addition to lifestyle modification with diet and exercise, most patients in the high-risk group will require pharmacotherapy (Table 4.1) with statins.[3-5]

PHARMACOTHERAPY WITH STATINS IN THE TREATMENT OF HIGH LDL-C

- HMG-CoA reductase inhibitors (statins) are the agents of choice for LDL-C lowering. A statin-induced reduction in LDL-C decreases the risk of coronary heart disease (CHD) and all-cause mortality in people at a high risk of CHD. The relative risk reduction is similar in men and women for both middle-aged and elderly people.

BOX 4.1
Diet and Lifestyle Changes in the Prevention of Coronary Artery Disease

CARDIAC REHABILITATION

- Cardiac rehabilitation is an important, professionally supervised program usually lasting between 6 and 10 weeks; it is a critical step on the road to recovery from a heart attack.
- Cardiac rehabilitation programs include physical activity, health education, counselling, behaviour modification strategies and support for self-management.

DIET

- Healthy eating pattern include:
  - mainly plant-based food: vegetables, fruits (five servings of vegetables and two of fruit daily), nuts, seeds, legumes, wholegrain breads, pasta, rice, potatoes, herbs and spices
  - moderate amounts of: low-fat or reduced-fat dairy products, polyunsaturated and monounsaturated fats (olive oil, canola oil)
  - several times a week: fish and seafood, poultry, eggs
  - less often: moderate amounts of lean, unprocessed meats, sweets.

OTHER

- At least 30 minutes of moderate-intensity physical activity is recommended most days of the week. Patients with chronic conditions may need to be referred to an exercise physiologist or to a physiotherapist.
- Weight reduction for patients with body mass index (BMI) more than 25 kg/m². Patients with central obesity aim to reduce waist measurement to less than 94 cm for men and less than 80 cm for women (Asian men <90 cm).
- Smoking cessation: consider nicotine replacement therapy in patients who smoke more than 10 cigarettes per day.
- Wine in moderation: limit alcohol intake less than two standard drinks per day for men, less than one standard drink per day for women and no more than four on any occasion.
- Patients (especially those with a history of hypertension/heart failure) should limit salt intake to less than 4 g/day. There is strong evidence that salt restriction can reduce systolic blood pressure by approximately 4–5 mmHg in hypertensive patients and 2 mmHg in normotensive individuals.

TABLE 4.1 Dyslipidaemia	
Low-density lipoprotein cholesterol (LDL-C)	• LDL-C remains the primary target of lipid-altering therapies. • HMG-CoA reductase inhibitors (statins) are the agents of choice for LDL-C lowering. • Commonly prescribed statins at recommended doses typically reduce LDL-C levels by 30%–45%. • Ezetimibe reduces absorption of cholesterol from the intestine. Its addition to statin therapy lowers LDL-C by approximately 24%. • The PCSK9 inhibitor evolocumab lowers LDL-C levels by 59% compared with placebo. • Despite the fact that there is a clear beneficial effect on the HDL-C concentration and an improvement in TG concentration, exercise training has no significant effect on the total cholesterol or LDL-C concentrations.
High-density lipoprotein cholesterol (HDL-C)	• There is a consistent linear association between weight loss and HDL-C concentrations in both men and women. For every 3 kg of weight loss, HDL-C levels increase by 1 mg/dL when weight reduction is maintained.[4] • Regular exercise is associated with increased levels of HDL-C. • Alcohol increases HDL-C level in a dose-dependent manner. • Drugs that increase HDL-C levels include niacin, fibrates and statins. Among lipid-modifying agents, niacin is the most potent agent currently available to increase HDL-C. • Niacin increases HDL-C by 15%–35% and fibrate increases it by 10%–15%. • Statins have been considered to have only a modest effect on raising HDL-C, with most studies showing a <10% increase in HDL-C concentrations.[5]
Triglyceride (TG)	• TG levels are markedly affected by body weight and fat distribution. Weight loss and a healthy Mediterranean diet with replacement of some dietary carbohydrate with unsaturated fat may reduce TG by 10%–20%. • Exercise is effective in lowering TGs, especially when baseline levels are elevated and total caloric intake is also reduced. • Fibrate, niacin and omega-3 are effective in reducing TG production by 20%–50%. • Overall, statins reduce TG levels in the range of 10%–20%.

- LDL-C remains the primary target of lipid-altering therapies. The beneficial effects of statins on CHD and total mortality appear to be directly proportional to the degree to which lipids are lowered. A 1.0 mmol/L reduction in plasma total cholesterol translates into a 23% reduction in the risk of future coronary events. Commonly prescribed statins at recommended doses typically reduce LDL-C levels by 30%–45%.

- PCSK9 (proprotein convertase subtilisin/kexin type 9) inhibitors are monoclonal antibodies that bind plasma PCSK9, directing more LDL, recycling towards the hepatic surface and effectively lowering plasma LDL-C. Recently, the randomised, double-blind, placebo-controlled FOURIER trial[6] showed that, in patients with atherosclerotic cardiovascular disease and LDL-C levels of 1.8 mmol/L or higher who were receiving statin therapy, inhibition of PCSK9 with evolocumab lowered LDL-C levels by 59% compared with placebo. There was a 15% reduction in the risk of the primary composite end point of cardiovascular death, myocardial infarction, stroke, hospitalisation for unstable angina, or coronary revascularisation over 3 years follow-up. Evolocumab is estimated to cost approximately US$14,350 per patient for a 1-year supply in the United States, or approximately $1200 per month (it is subsidised in Australia for treatment of familial homozygous hypercholesterolaemia).

- Ezetimibe reduces absorption of cholesterol from the intestine. In the IMPROVE-IT trial,[7] the addition of ezetimibe to statin therapy lowered LDL-C by approximately 24%. The combination of simvastatin and ezetimibe also resulted in a significantly lower risk of cardiovascular events than statin monotherapy.

- All adults at high risk should have lipid levels monitored every 6–12 months, or at a minimum annually, as part of an ongoing assessment and management of overall cardiovascular disease (CVD) risk.

Who Needs a Statin?

- Statin therapy is recommended for all people with clinical evidence of vascular disease (such as CHD, stroke or peripheral arterial disease) and should be commenced in hospital for those admitted with ACS with an aim to achieve a total cholesterol of <4 and an LDL-C <1.8 mmol/L.
- The current Australian guideline recommends the use of 5-year absolute cardiovascular risk calculator to assess future risks.[8] Statin use for primary prevention of cardiovascular disease (CVD) is considered in the high-risk patient category. The following patients who are considered 'high risk of CVD' does not require CVD risk calculation:
  - diabetes and age > 60 years
  - diabetes with microalbuminuria
  - moderate or severe chronic kidney disease
  - previous diagnosis of familial hypercholesterolaemia
  - systolic blood pressure ≥180 mmHg or diastolic blood pressure ≥110 mmHg
  - serum total cholesterol >7.5 mmol/L.
- In addition, people with familial hypercholesterolaemia and a high absolute risk (more than 2.5% per year) should be considered for statin therapy. There is additional benefit to be gained from the progressive lowering of cholesterol levels with no apparent lower limit.
- Compared with the general population in the United States, the prevalence of CHD in Asian Indians is approximately four times higher and remains a leading cause of death.[9] The consequences of atherosclerosis in the Asian Indian populations tend to be more severe and develop earlier in life. Although total cholesterol and LDL-C levels are similar to whites, HDL levels are lower, TG levels are higher and those of other lipoproteins such as lipoprotein (a) are also higher. Aggressive statin therapy can significantly lower LDL-C levels, modestly decrease TGs and elevate HDL-C and thereby stabilise atherosclerotic plaques. Since statins were first approved in 1987, their ability to reduce the risks of vascular death, non-fatal MI, stroke and the need for arterial revascularisation has been shown in several large, high-quality randomised trials in both primary and secondary prevention.[9]

Goals of Lipid Lowering in Patients With Vascular Disease

- Recent trials have demonstrated the benefit of lowering LDL-C to levels substantially below the previously recommended target in high-risk patients with existing CHD. The results of these trials support a target LDL-C of <1.8 mmol/L for this patient population. There is additional benefit from progressive lowering of cholesterol levels, with no apparent lower limit.
- Most guidelines put increased emphasis on benefits of statins for all patients with vascular disease regardless of LDL-C level.[8]

Safety of Statin Treatment

- Statins are well tolerated and safe. The most common adverse effect is muscular aches, followed by mildly altered liver function tests. Myopathy, or muscle pain or weakness, with blood creatine kinase (CK) levels more than 10 times the upper limit of normal is called rhabdomyolysis; it typically occurs in fewer than 1 in 10,000 patients receiving standard statin doses and requires statin therapy to be stopped.
- Adverse effects on the liver are rare at standard statin doses. All statins are associated with asymptomatic increases in concentrations of liver transaminases but this is not clearly associated with increased risk for liver disease. Both myopathy and rhabdomyolysis occur more often with higher statin doses and are reversed by stopping statin use, usually leading to full recovery.[8]
- For patients with statin side effects, lower doses, alternative statins and alternate-day dosing should be trialled wherever possible. If more-potent statins or higher doses are not tolerated, adding ezetimibe to low-dose statins is also an option.

Role of Statin in Reducing the Atheroma Volume

Intensive statin therapy not only prevents the progression of coronary atherosclerosis but can also lead to plaque regression or stabilisation. 'ASTEROID' – a study to evaluate the effect of rosuvastatin on intravascular ultrasound-derived coronary atheroma burden – showed that very intensive cholesterol lowering with rosuvastatin resulted in significant regression of atherosclerosis as measured by intravascular ultrasound.[10] The results also demonstrated that no apparent LDL-C 'threshold' exists beyond which the benefits of LDL-C reduction no longer apply. To achieve regression, lower is better. Similarly, the REVERSAL trial supported these findings.[11]

Efficacy of Different Statins in Prevention of Vascular Disease

- All statins lower LDL-C levels but have different potency at approved dosages. The STELLAR trial[12] compared the degree of LDL-C lowering and HDL-C raising achieved with four different statins. The drugs differed in potency at comparable dosages and were ranked in the following order, from greater to lesser: rosuvastatin, atorvastatin, simvastatin, pravastatin.

- If LDL-C goals are not achieved, consider switching to a more potent statin. Generally, 10 mg of rosuvastatin, 20 mg of atorvastatin, 40 mg of simvastatin and 80 mg of pravastatin have equivalent LDL-C-lowering capacity.

WHAT ARE THE ROLES OF DIFFERENT ANTIPLATELET MEDICATIONS?

- Aspirin (100–150 mg/day) should be continued indefinitely unless it is not tolerated or an indication for a different anticoagulation becomes apparent.
- Dual-antiplatelet therapy with aspirin and a P2Y12 inhibitor (ticagrelor, prasugrel or clopidogrel) should be prescribed for up to 12 months in patients with ACS, regardless of whether coronary revascularisation was performed.

Aspirin

- Aspirin, or acetylsalicylic acid (ASA), inhibits thromboxane A_2 synthesis by irreversibly acetylating cyclooxygenase-1 in platelets and megakaryocytes.
- Platelets are unable to regenerate cyclooxygenase, hence the immediate antithrombotic effect of ASA remains for the lifespan of the platelet (8–10 days).
- Aspirin reduces the risk of serious vascular events in high-risk patients by about 23% and is recommended as the first-line antiplatelet drug. Some adverse effects of aspirin include:
  - It can cause non-fatal extra cranial haemorrhage (1–2 per 1000 patients treated per year).
  - There is an increased risk of intracranial haemorrhage of about 1 per 1000 patients when treated for 3 years.
  - ASA is directly ulcerogenic as it suppresses gastric mucosal prostaglandin synthesis. One in 10 patients taking it will have an endoscopically proven ulcer at 28 days.[13]

Clopidogrel

- Clopidogrel is metabolised in the liver into active compounds which covalently bind to the adenosine diphosphate (ADP) receptors on platelets and dramatically reduce platelet activation. An oral loading dose of 300–600 mg of clopidogrel produces detectable inhibition of ADP-induced platelet aggregation after 2 hours (max after 6 hours).

- Severe neutropenia has been noted in 0.1% of patients. Rarely, thrombotic thrombocytopenic purpura has also been reported with the use of clopidogrel.
- Clopidogrel and ASA caused a 20% relative risk reduction (stroke, MI or vascular death) compared with ASA alone, at the expense of 10 extra cases of cranial bleeding per 1000 patients treated, in a group of patients following a NSTEMI with 9 months of follow-up.
- Treatment with ASA and clopidogrel for 12 months following percutaneous transluminal coronary angioplasty (PTCA) caused a 27% relative risk reduction (stroke, MI or vascular death) compared with ASA alone.[14,15]
- In the past, the mainstay of antiplatelet therapy for patients with ACS, including those undergoing early percutaneous coronary intervention, has been the combination of aspirin and clopidogrel. However, clopidogrel has several potential limitations that led to the search for newer antiplatelet agents. The onset of action of clopidogrel is delayed, with a 'therapeutic' level of 50% inhibition of ADP-induced platelet aggregation being reached only 4–6 hours after a 300 mg loading dose, and 2 hours after a 600 mg dose.[1]

Ticagrelor

- Ticagrelor is a potent, reversibly binding, direct-acting P2Y12 receptor antagonist that provides faster, greater and more consistent P2Y12 inhibition than does clopidogrel.
- The PLATO study[16] showed that treatment with ticagrelor, as compared with clopidogrel, in patients with acute coronary syndromes with or without ST-segment elevation significantly reduced the rate of death (a relative reduction of 22% in the rate of death from any cause at 1 year), MI or stroke. The benefits with ticagrelor were seen regardless of whether invasive or non-invasive management was planned.
- The ticagrelor and clopidogrel groups did not differ significantly with regard to the rates of major bleeding as defined in the trial. Dyspnoea was more common in the ticagrelor group than in the clopidogrel group (in 13.8% of patients vs 7.8%).[16]

Prasugrel

- Prasugrel is a third-generation thienopyridine, an ADP receptor antagonist that is a potent inhibitor of platelet activation and aggregation. A benefit of prasugrel is its rapid onset of action. Because of this it can be given immediately prior to stenting, once the coronary anatomy is confirmed and it is determined that urgent bypass surgery is not required.

Within a short time period it reaches concentrations in the blood significant enough to inhibit platelet functions and decrease the risk of stent thrombosis. The prasugrel active metabolite concentration peaks in the plasma at 30 minutes.[3]

- Prasugrel co-administered with aspirin is indicated for the prevention of atherothrombotic events (MI, stroke and cardiovascular death) in patients with acute coronary syndromes (moderate- to high-risk unstable angina (UA), NSTEMI or STEMI) who are to undergo percutaneous coronary intervention (PCI).
- The pharmacokinetic and pharmacodynamic superiority of prasugrel is translated into improved ischaemic outcomes but more bleeding in patients with ACS and planned PCI.

Summary of Dual Antiplatelet Agents

Use of ticagrelor is advised among a broad spectrum of ACS patients with STEMI or NSTEMI who are at an intermediate to high risk of an ischaemic event in the absence of atrioventricular (AV) conduction disorders (second- and third-degree AV block) and asthma/chronic obstructive pulmonary disease (COPD). Clopidogrel is recommended for patients who cannot receive ticagrelor or prasugrel, as an adjunctive agent with fibrinolysis or for those requiring oral anticoagulation.

ROLE OF BETA-BLOCKERS AND ACE INHIBITORS IN SECONDARY PREVENTION OF CARDIOVASCULAR DISEASE
Beta-Blockers[17,18]

- Beta-blockers have been used extensively in the past after acute myocardial infarction (AMI) as part of secondary prevention. The evidence for beta-blocker therapy post-AMI is based largely on results of trials conducted before the current revascularisation, dual-antiplatelet and statin practice era.
- Extrapolating from pre-reperfusion-era trials, patients presenting late with large infarct size and perhaps without revascularisation may have the greatest benefit from continuation of oral beta-blockers, including a potential reduction in mortality and sudden death. These are also patients who will have reduced left ventricular ejection fraction (LVEF) where beta-blockers remain the standard of care. Current guidelines recommend treatment with vasodilatory beta-blockers (e.g. carvedilol, bisoprolol, nebivolol and metoprolol succinate) in patients with LVEF <40% unless contraindicated.
- However, there remains no clear consensus regarding the appropriate role and duration of treatment with

beta-blockers in post-AMI patients with normal LVEF who have been fully revascularised and are not experiencing angina or arrhythmias.
- A recent meta-analysis of beta-blocker use after MI sought to explore the effect of contemporary treatment (i.e. reperfusion, aspirin and statins) on the benefits of beta-blocker use and clinical outcomes in patients with MI. Sixty randomised controlled trials were included, with 102,003 patients stratified into pre-reperfusion-era or reperfusion-era trials with the primary outcome of all-cause mortality. Interestingly, beta-blocker use in the pre-reperfusion era was associated with reduced all-cause mortality at 30 days (risk ratio (RR) 0.87; 95% CI, 0.79, 0.96) and even after 1 year (RR 0.91; 95% CI, 0.66, 0.98). In the reperfusion era, on the other hand, there was no change in sudden death or mortality.

Angiotensin Converting Enzyme (ACE) Inhibitors/Angiotensin Receptor Blockers (ARBs)

- ACE inhibitors and ARBs are the most commonly used drugs to provide therapeutic modulation of angiotensin II. Both ACE inhibitors and ARBs attenuate the effects of angiotensin II, but through different mechanisms – ACE inhibitors reduce the synthesis of angiotensin II, whereas ARBs bind to angiotensin II type 1 (AT1) receptors to block their activation.
- Current guidelines recommend the initiation and continuation of ACE inhibitors or ARBs in patients with evidence of heart failure, left ventricular systolic dysfunction, diabetes, anterior MI or co-existing hypertension.
- In EUROPA trial patients with coronary artery disease, ACE inhibitor therapy was shown to significantly reduce the risk of MI and cardiovascular death. Results from the EUROPA trial suggests that the reduction in cardiovascular events was greater than what would be expected from the reduction in blood pressure alone.[19]

John successfully finished cardiac rehabilitation and stopped smoking. He was adherent to all prescribed medications and living a healthy active lifestyle. He lost 8 kg intentionally and went back to work as a truck driver (see Table 4.2).

John was re-admitted to the hospital 2 years later again with chest pain. He was found to be in atrial fibrillation with ECG showing lateral ST depression and a troponin rise.

His angiogram showed new 80% stenosis in the left circumflex artery (LCX). Urgent angioplasty was performed with a drug-eluting stent to the LCX.

TABLE 4.2
Driving After Myocardial Infarction

Minimum Non-Driving Period Following a Cardiac Event/Procedure	Private Vehicle Drivers	Commercial Vehicle Drivers
ISCHAEMIC HEART DISEASE		
Acute myocardial infarction	2 weeks	4 weeks
Percutaneous coronary intervention	2 days	4 weeks
Coronary artery bypass grafts	4 weeks	3 months
Disorders of rate, rhythm and conduction		
Cardiac arrest	6 months	6 months
Implantable cardioverter defibrillator (ICD) insertion	6 months after cardiac arrest	Not eligible to hold a commercial licence
Generator change of an ICD	2 weeks	Not applicable
ICD therapy associated with symptoms of haemodynamic compromise	4 weeks	Not applicable
Cardiac pacemaker insertion	2 weeks	4 weeks
OTHER		
Valvular replacement (including treatment with mitral clips and transcutaneous aortic valve replacement)	4 weeks	3 months
Syncope (due to cardiovascular cause)	4 weeks	3 months
Deep vein thrombosis	2 weeks	2 weeks
Pulmonary embolism	6 weeks	6 weeks

(Modified from *Assessing fitness to drive 2016* as amended up to August 2017, ISBN: 978-1-925451-95-5, Austroads Publication Number: AP-G56-17.)

MANAGEMENT OF CORONARY ARTERY DISEASE IN THE PRESENCE OF ATRIAL FIBRILLATION

- Patients with a history of atrial fibrillation taking an anticoagulant requiring elective stenting, or presenting with acute coronary syndromes, usually require antiplatelet agents. The composition and duration of antiplatelet treatment and anticoagulation depends on a careful balancing of the risk of thrombosis and the risk of bleeding.
- For elective angioplasty for coronary disease, current guidelines recommend 1 month of triple therapy, generally with either a reduced dose of oral anticoagulant (15 mg of rivaroxaban daily or 110 mg twice daily dabigatran or 2.5 mg twice daily of apixaban) in combination with aspirin and clopidogrel, followed by dual therapy (an oral anticoagulant plus a single antiplatelet agent with either aspirin or clopidogrel) for up to 6–12 months, depending on bleeding risk,

with continuation of oral anticoagulant monotherapy thereafter.
- For angioplasty in the setting of ACS, the ESC guidelines recommend either 1 month or 6 months of triple therapy in the high- and low-bleeding risk groups (HAS-BLED score above 3 or between 0 and 2 – see Fig. 12.4) respectively, followed by dual therapy for the remainder of the 12-month period.[20]

Role of Double Therapy vs Triple Therapy

- Though 'triple therapy' offers the best protection against thrombosis, it also increases the risk of bleeding significantly. A number of recent trials have shown that 'double therapy' with an oral anticoagulant and single antiplatelet agent reduces risk of bleeding significantly but, unfortunately, none of the trials clearly gives us the answer as to whether the risk of thrombosis is increased with omission of aspirin.
- An open-label, multicentre, randomised controlled trial, assessing the use of clopidogrel with or without

aspirin in patients taking oral anticoagulant therapy (warfarin) and undergoing percutaneous coronary intervention, found that the use of clopidogrel without aspirin is associated with a significant reduction in bleeding complications and no increase in the rate of thrombotic events.[21]

- The PIONEER AF-PCI trial was the first prospective study in patients with atrial fibrillation undergoing percutaneous angioplasty (PCI) to compare low-dose rivaroxaban regimens plus a P2Y12 inhibitor (clopidogrel) for 12 months with initial therapy with warfarin (target INR 2.0–3.0) plus dual antiplatelet agents, followed by warfarin and aspirin. The trial demonstrated that rivaroxaban-based treatment regimens were associated with reduced rates of clinically significant bleeding events compared with the warfarin-based regimen.[22]

- In the RE-DUAL PCI trial, which enrolled patients with atrial fibrillation who had undergone percutaneous coronary angioplasty, the risk of bleeding was found to be lower among those who received dual therapy with dabigatran and a P2Y12 inhibitor (clopidogrel or ticagrelor) than among those who received triple therapy with warfarin, a P2Y12 inhibitor and aspirin. Dual therapy was not inferior to triple therapy with respect to the risk of thromboembolic events.[23]

- Similarly, in the more-recent AUGUSTUS trial, patients with atrial fibrillation and a recent (14 days after) ACS or PCI treated with a P2Y12 inhibitor were randomised to antithrombotic regimen with either warfarin or apixaban, with or without aspirin. An antithrombotic regimen that included apixaban and a P2Y12 inhibitor without aspirin resulted in less bleeding and fewer hospitalisations. Unfortunately, the trial was underpowered for assessing coronary ischaemic events.[24]

REFERENCES

1. Kraus WE, Houmard JA, Duscha BD, Knetzger KJ, Wharton MB, McCartney JS, et al. Effects of the amount and intensity of exercise on plasma lipoproteins. *N Engl J Med* 2002;**347**:1483–92.
2. Moffatt RJ. Effects of cessation of smoking on serum lipids and high density lipoprotein-cholesterol. *Atherosclerosis* 1988;**74**(1–2):85–9.
3. Estruch R, Ros E, Salas-Salvadó J, Covas MI, Corella D, Arós F, et al. Retraction and republication: primary prevention of cardiovascular disease with a Mediterranean diet. *N Engl J Med* 2018;**368**:1279–90.
4. Dattilo AM, Kris-Etherton PM. Effects of weight reduction on blood lipids and lipoproteins: a meta-analysis. *Am J Clin Nutr* 1992;**56**:320–8.
5. Belalcazar LM, Ballantyne CM. Defining specific goals of therapy in treating dyslipidemia in the patient with low high-density lipoprotein cholesterol. *Prog Cardiovasc Dis* 1998;**41**:151–74.
6. Sabatine MS, Giugliano RP, Keech AC, Honarpour N, Wiviott SD, Murphy SA, et al; FOURIER Steering Committee and Investigators. Evolocumab and clinical outcomes in patients with cardiovascular disease. *N Engl J Med* 2017;**376**(18):1713–22.
7. Cannon CP, Blazing MA, Giugliano RP, McCagg A, White JA, Theroux P, et al. IMPROVE-IT Investigators. Ezetimibe added to statin therapy after acute coronary syndromes. *N Engl J Med* 2015;**372**:2387–97.
8. National Heart Foundation of Australia and the Cardiac Society of Australia and New Zealand. *Lipid management guidelines 2018.* https://www.heartfoundation.org.au/images/uploads/publications/Absolute-CVD-Risk-Quick-Reference-Guide_2018.pdf.
9. Enas EA, Yusuf S, Mehta JL. Prevalence of coronary artery disease in Asian Indians. *Am J Cardiol* 1992;**70**:945–9.
10. Nissen SE, Nicholls SJ, Sipahi I, Libby P, Raichlen JS, Ballantyne CM, et al; ASTEROID Investigators. Effect of very high-intensity statin therapy on regression of coronary atherosclerosis: the ASTEROID trial. *JAMA* 2006;**295**(13):1556–65.
11. Stegman B, Shao M, Nicholls SJ, Elshazly M, Cho L, King P, et al. Coronary atheroma progression rates in men and women following high-intensity statin therapy: a pooled analysis of REVERSAL, ASTEROID and SATURN. *Atherosclerosis* 2016;**254**:78–84.
12. KcKenney JM. Comparison of the efficacy of rosuvastatin versus atorvastatin, simvastatin, and pravastatin in achieving lipid goals: results from the STELLAR trial. *Curr Med Res Opin* 2003;**19**(8):689–98.
13. Antithrombotic Trialists' Collaboration. Collaborative meta-analysis of randomised trials of antiplatelet therapy for prevention of death, myocardial infarction, and stroke in high risk patients. *BMJ* 2002;**324**:71–86.
14. Steinhubi SR, Berger PB, Mann JT 3rd, Fry ET, DeLago A, Wilmer C, et al; CREDO Investigators. Clopidogrel for the Reduction of Events During Observation. Early and sustained dual oral antiplatelet therapy following percutaneous coronary intervention: a randomized controlled trial. *JAMA* 2002;**288**:2411–20.
15. Yusuf S, Zhao F, Mehta SR, Chrolavicius S, Tognoni G, Fox KK, Clopidogrel in Unstable Angina to Prevent Recurrent Events Trial Investigators. Effects of clopidogrel in addition to aspirin in patients with acute coronary syndromes without ST-segment elevation. *N Engl J Med* 2001;**345**:494–502.
16. Wallentin L, Becker RC, Budaj A, Cannon CP, Emanuelsson H, Held C, Freij A, et al; PLATO Investigators. Ticagrelor versus clopidogrel in patients with acute coronary syndromes. *N Engl J Med* 2009;**361**:1045–57.
17. Smith SC Jr, Benjamin EJ, Bonow RO, Braun LT, Creager MA, Franklin BA, et al; World Heart Federation and the Preventive Cardiovascular Nurses Association. AHA/ACCF secondary prevention and risk reduction therapy for patients with

coronary and other atherosclerotic vascular disease: 2011 update: a guideline from the American Heart Association and American College of Cardiology Foundation. *Circulation* 2011;**124**:2458–73.

18. Bangalore S, Makani H, Radford M, Thakur K, Toklu B, Katz SD, et al. Clinical outcomes with μ-blockers for myocardial infarction: a meta-analysis of randomized trials. *Am J Med* 2014;**127**:939–53.

19. Fox KM, EURopean trial On reduction of cardiac events with Perindopril in stable coronary Artery disease investigators. Efficacy of perindopril in reduction of cardiovascular events among patients with stable coronary artery disease: randomised, double-blind, placebo-controlled, multicentre trial (the EUROPA study). *Lancet* 2003;**362**(9386):782–8.

20. Kirchhof P, Benussi S, Kotecha D, Ahlsson A, Atar D, Casadei B, et al; ESC Scientific Document Group. 2016 ESC Guidelines for the management of atrial fibrillation. *Eur Heart J* 2016;**37**(38):2893–962.

21. Dewilde WJ, Oirbans T, Verheugt FW, Kelder JC, De Smet BJ, Herrman JP, et al; WOEST study investigators. Use of clopidogrel with or without aspirin in patients taking oral anticoagulant therapy and undergoing percutaneous coronary intervention: an open-label, randomised, controlled trial. *Lancet* 2013;**381**(9872):1107–15.

22. Gibson CM, Mehran R, Bode C, Halperin J, Verheugt FW, Wildgoose P, et al. Prevention of bleeding in patients with atrial fibrillation undergoing PCI. *N Engl J Med* 2016;**375**(25):2423–34.

23. Cannon CP, Bhatt DL, Oldgren J, Lip GYH, Ellis SG, Kimura T, et al; RE-DUAL PCI Steering Committee and Investigators. Dual antithrombotic therapy with dabigatran after PCI in atrial fibrillation. *N Engl J Med* 2017;**377**:1513–24.

24. Lopes RD, Heizer G, Aronson R, Vora AN, Massaro T, Mehran R, et al; AUGUSTUS Investigators. Antithrombotic therapy after acute coronary syndrome or PCI in atrial fibrillation. *N Engl J Med* 2019;**380**(16):1509–24.

Management of Acute Chest Pain

CASE 7 SCENARIO: DAWN WITH CHEST PAIN

68-year-old Dawn presents to the hospital emergency with severe intermittent chest pain. The pain started 4 hours previously. She is a smoker and takes amlodipine 10 mg daily for hypertension. She does not have other traditional risk factors for vascular disease. The examination and initial ECG are unremarkable. Currently she is pain free.

Question
A true statement about Dawn's chest pain includes:
1. *The differential diagnosis of chest pain could include 'acute coronary syndrome'.*
2. *Serial ECGs should be done every 10–15 minutes until Dawn is pain free.*
3. *Dawn should have blood tests including serial troponins (cTnI).*
4. *Based on her ECG, she could be considered for immediate thrombolysis.*
5. *She should be referred for coronary angiography.*

DIFFERENTIAL DIAGNOSIS OF CHEST PAIN

Chest pain is a common presenting symptom in the emergency department. It has a variety of differential diagnoses including a number of serious, life-threatening conditions. Most of the following conditions may produce non-specific ECG changes and a positive troponin test,

adding diagnostic confusion and uncertainty. Consider potentially life-threatening causes of chest pain and evaluate the need for emergency care before considering other common causes of chest pain.

LIFE-THREATENING CAUSES OF CHEST PAIN IN THE EMERGENCY DEPARTMENT
Acute Coronary Syndrome
The term acute coronary syndrome (ACS) refers to a spectrum of conditions compatible with acute myocardial ischaemia and / or infarction that are usually caused by an abrupt reduction in coronary blood flow. These conditions include unstable angina, ST-segment elevation myocardial infarction (STEMI) and non-ST elevation myocardial infarction (NSTEMI) (Fig. 5.1).

Aortic Dissection
- This is a relatively rare condition which can be difficult to diagnose. A high index of suspicion is necessary for the diagnosis to be made.
- Patients with aortic dissections most commonly describe a sudden, severe tearing pain radiating through to the back.
- Patients are often hypertensive. Neurological deficits can be a presenting sign in up to 20% of cases. A blood pressure difference between the two arms of greater than 20 mmHg should increase the suspicion of aortic dissection.

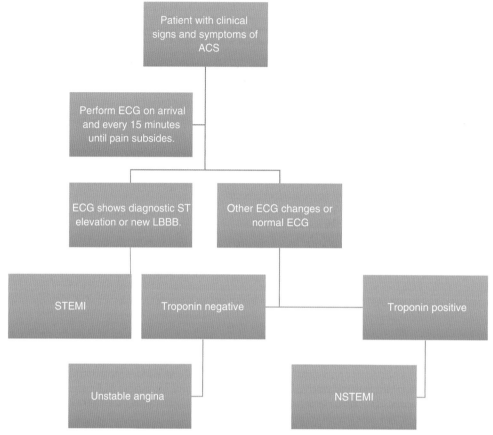

FIG. 5.1 Classification of acute coronary syndrome (ACS). LBBB=left bundle branch block; NSTEMI=non-ST elevation myocardial infarction; STEMI=ST-segment elevation myocardial infarction.

- Chest x-ray abnormalities are common and include a widened mediastinum. A bedside echocardiogram, particularly a transoesophageal echocardiogram, can be very useful. CT scanning, especially with arterial contrast enhancement, is the investigation of choice. It has high sensitivity and specificity.

Pulmonary Embolism

- Pulmonary embolism (PE) can present with pleuritic chest pain (66%), dyspnoea (73%), cough (37%) or haemoptysis (13%).
- Risk factors associated with PE include recent surgery, trauma or travel with a history of immobilisation, malignancy, past history of deep vein thrombosis (DVT) or PE and hypercoagulable states. The majority of patients with PE presents with the sudden onset of pleuritic chest pain or shortness of breath. Other presentations can include syncope and haemoptysis.

- The physical examination is usually non-specific; however, an unexplained tachycardia, or signs of a DVT or congestive cardiac failure, may indicate the presence of a PE. Other findings can include tachypnoea.
- The ECG is frequently abnormal but non-specific. The most common finding is sinus tachycardia. Other ECG findings suggestive of PE include right (R) bundle branch block, T-wave inversion in V1–3 and a S1Q3T3 pattern.
- The D-dimer test is useful for excluding PE in patients who are of low or intermediate risk (a highly sensitive test with low false-negative rate). Unfortunately, D-dimer has low specificity (a high false-positive rate).
- A normal chest x-ray (CXR) in a patient with hypoxia is suggestive of a PE. CT pulmonary angiography or VQ scanning is indicated in patients who are of low

or intermediate risk with positive D-dimers or in patients who are at high risk.

- Echocardiography is useful in suspected PE. It may show right heart dilation; increased right ventricular systolic pressure and dysfunction and sometimes a large thrombus may be visible in the main pulmonary artery.

Tension Pneumothorax

- Symptoms of chest pain are usually sudden in onset, localised to the side of the pneumothorax and pleuritic in nature. Dyspnoea is also common.
- The classic examination findings are reduced or absent breath sounds and hyper-resonance on percussion on the affected side.
- In a patient with suspected pneumothorax, the chest x-ray is the investigation of choice.

Ruptured Oesophagus

- The classic presentation of spontaneous oesophageal rupture is severe vomiting or retching followed by acute, severe chest or epigastric pain.
- There may be subcutaneous emphysema on the chest wall.

EPIDEMIOLOGY OF CHEST PAIN IN PRIMARY CARE AND EMERGENCY DEPARTMENT SETTINGS[1]

- Musculoskeletal, including costochondritis 36%
- Gastrointestinal 19%
- Cardiac 16%, stable angina 10.5%, unstable angina or MI 1.5%
- Other cardiac 3.8%
- Psychiatric 8%
- Pulmonary 5%
- Other/unknown 16%

TYPICAL/ATYPICAL SYMPTOMS

Although the history of presenting symptoms is very important in diagnosing ACS, it lacks both sensitivity and specificity. Typical ischaemic-type chest pain has been described as deep, poorly localised chest pain or discomfort, pressure, tightness or heaviness. The pain may radiate to the neck, jaw, shoulders, back or arms.

Patients Frequently Presenting With Atypical Symptoms[2]

Women, elderly patients, patients with dementia and those with diabetes may not describe typical ischaemic-sounding chest pain. In addition, patients with distractive pain (e.g. a concurrent hip fracture) may underestimate or not report chest pain. The diagnosis of MI should be considered with presenting symptoms termed 'angina equivalents', especially in the above groups of patients.

Angina Equivalents

These can include but are not limited to:

- isolated unexplained new-onset or worsened exertional dyspnoea – the most common angina-equivalent symptom, especially in older patients
- any discomfort or pain between the umbilicus and the mouth (including epigastric pain or indigestion-like symptoms)
- exertional throat pain or pain in the arms, more commonly in the medial aspect of the left arm
- less-common isolated presentations, primarily in older adults, including nausea, vomiting, diaphoresis, unexplained fatigue, dizziness and belching on exertion
- rarely do patients with ACS present with syncope as the primary symptom.

Features Not Characteristic of Myocardial Ischaemia

These include the following[2]:

- pleuritic pain (i.e. sharp or knifelike pain brought on by respiratory movements or cough)
- primary or sole location of discomfort in the middle or lower abdominal region
- pain that may be localised to the tip of one finger, particularly over the left ventricular apex or a costochondral junction
- pain reproduced with movement or palpation of the chest wall or arms
- very brief episodes of pain that last a few seconds
- pain that radiates into the lower extremities.

It is recommended that a patient with acute chest pain or other symptoms suggestive of an MI should receive a 12-lead ECG within 10 minutes. This initial assessment is to identify rapidly those patients with an acute STEMI for consideration of emergency reperfusion therapy if clinically indicated. In patients with ongoing chest pain and an unremarkable initial ECG, serial ECGs should be performed every 10–15 minutes to look for evidence of an evolving infarction.[3]

In NSTEMI there is no persistent ST-segment elevation or new left bundle branch block. ECG changes in these patients may include transient ST-segment elevation (<20 minutes), ST-segment depression or T-wave

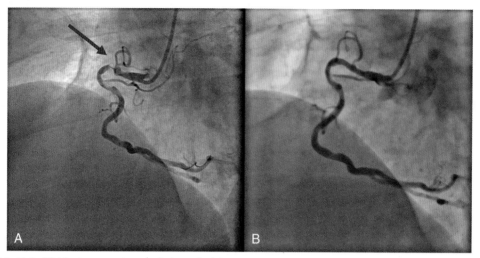

FIG. 5.2 **(A)** Ninety percent stenosis (arrow) of the tortuous proximal right coronary artery; **(B)** artery after stenting. NSTEMI is generally associated with white, platelet-rich partially occlusive thrombus.

changes. The ECG may be normal in about one-third of cases.

CARDIAC ENZYMES IN THE MANAGEMENT OF ACUTE CHEST PAIN[4]

- Cardiac troponin is a highly sensitive biomarker of myocardial injury which is used in the diagnosis of acute MI and for risk stratification of patients with acute coronary symptoms. In 2012, the third universal definition of myocardial infarction emphasised that elevations in biomarkers were fundamental to the diagnosis of acute MI.[4]
- The serum troponin level is very sensitive for detecting myocardial injury and indicates an adverse prognosis. However, troponin lacks specificity (a high false-positive rate) for the diagnosis of ACS as the troponin level is also elevated in a number of other conditions including sepsis, heart failure, renal failure, pulmonary embolism and pericarditis. (Type 1 MI from plaque rupture must be differentiated from type 2 MI from oxygen supply–demand imbalance in the context of another concurrent acute illness.) The test may be difficult to interpret when it is measured in patients who do not have chest pain.
- In general, an increased serum troponin level warrants further investigations and an expert opinion. While diagnosing MI, the third universal definition of MI should be considered rather than relying solely on troponin elevation.[4]

RISK STRATIFICATION IN PATIENTS WITH CHEST PAIN

- In contrast to STEMI, NSTEMI is generally associated with a white, platelet-rich, partially occlusive thrombus (Figs 5.2 and 5.3 left, upper panel), whereas STEMI is generally caused by an occlusive thrombus (Fig. 5.3 right, upper panel). The clinical spectrum of NSTEMI varies, and the treatment strategy, including the timing of coronary angiography and revascularisation, depends on risk assessment using common clinical risk assessment scores.
- Formal risk stratification allows quantification of the risk of complications in patients with chest pain for up to 30 days after presentation. High-risk patients with non-ST-segment elevation acute coronary syndrome (NSTEACS) should be treated with aggressive medical management (including aspirin, ticagrelor/clopidogrel, heparin/enoxaparin).
- More than 25% of patients with these high-risk features will have a confirmed diagnosis of ACS and should be referred for inpatient investigation, including coronary angiography.[5]
- Intermediate-risk patients with NSTEMI should undergo an accelerated diagnostic evaluation and further assessment to allow reclassification as low or high risk.[3]

Risk assessment scores and clinical prediction algorithms that use clinical history, physical examination, the ECG and cardiac troponin levels have been developed

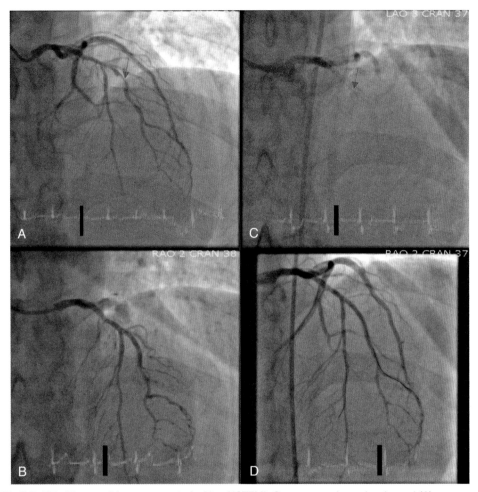

FIG. 5.3 This 56-year-old man presented with a NSTEMI. Coronary angiography showed **(A)** a bifurcation stenosis of the left anterior descending artery (LAD) and a large diagonal artery. The diagonal had an ulcerated plaque (arrow). Both arteries were stented using the culotte technique **(B)**. The patient presented 2 days later with chest pain and the ECG showed anterior STEMI. Angiography confirmed occlusion of the LAD and diagonal arteries **(C)** due to stent thrombosis. The arteries were re-opened using balloon angioplasty with a good angiographic result **(D)**.

to help identify patients with ACS at increased risk of an adverse outcome.[5]

TIMI AND GRACE SCORES

- Several scoring methods are commonly used to determine the risk of short-term and longer-term events in patients hospitalised with suspected ACS. The Thrombolysis in Myocardial Infarction (TIMI) score (Table 5.1)[6] and the Global Registry of Acute Coronary Events (GRACE) score are commonly known tools (Fig. 5.4).[7,8] The TIMI score is simple to use, but its discriminative accuracy is inferior to that of the GRACE score.
- The TIMI risk score uses seven variables in the scoring system including: age ≥65 years, three or more coronary artery disease (CAD) risk factors, known CAD, aspirin use in the past 7 days, severe angina (two or more episodes within 24 h), ST change ≥0.5 mm and positive cardiac marker.

- To calculate the score, a value of 1 is assigned when each variable was present and 0 when it was absent.

Historical	Points
Age ≥65	1
≥ 3 CAD risk factors	1
Known CAD (stenosis ≥ 50%)	1
ASA use in past 7 days	1
PRESENTATION	
Recent (≤24H) severe angina	1
↑ cardiac markers	1
ST deviation ≥ 0.5 mm	1
RISK SCORE = Total Points (0–7)	

RISK OF CARDIAC EVENTS (%)
BY 14 DAYS IN TIMI 11B*

Risk Score	Death or MI	Death, MI or Urgent Revasc
0/1	3	5
2	3	8
3	5	13
4	7	20
5	12	26
6/7	19	41

For more infor go to www.timi.org
*Entry criteria UA or NSTEMII defined as ischemic pain at rest within past 24H, with evidence of CAD (ST segment deviation or +marker)
(Reproduced with permission from Antman EM, Cohen Mk, Bernink PJLM, McCabe CH, Horacek T, Papuchis G, et al. The TIMI risk score for unstable angina/non-ST elevation MI. *JAMA* 2000;284:835–42.)

- The GRACE risk score predicts in-hospital mortality after ACS and includes the risk factors of age, Killip class, systolic blood pressure, ST-segment deviation, cardiac arrest during presentation, serum creatinine level, elevated troponin, and heart rate; it is available online and can be downloaded to portable electronic devices at: https://www.outcomes-umassmed.org/risk_models_grace_orig.aspx.
- Although both these indices are quite helpful in predicting the extent of the disease, the Global Registry showed a better performance and is more strongly associated with multivessel and left main coronary artery disease.

PARENTERAL ANTICOAGULANT THERAPY IN PATIENTS WITH ACS

In addition to antiplatelet therapy (discussed in Chapter 4), anticoagulation is recommended for all patients irrespective of initial treatment strategy.

Treatment options include: low-molecular-weight heparin (LMWH) (enoxaparin), fondaparinux, bivalirudin and unfractionated heparin (UFH).

Enoxaparin

- Enoxaparin is an LMWH that inhibits factor Xa, has a more predictable dose and is less likely than other agents to cause heparin-induced thrombocytopenia (HIT). The anticoagulant activity of LMWH does not require routine monitoring. The standard recommended dose of enoxaparin is 1 mg/kg subcutaneously every 12 hours, continued for the duration of hospitalisation or until PCI is performed. In patients with creatinine clearance <30 mL/min, there is a need to adjust the dose to 1 mg/kg subcutaneously once daily.

Fondaparinux

- Fondaparinux is a synthetic pentasaccharide that selectively binds reversibly to antithrombin and causes rapid and predictable inhibition of factor Xa. It has 100% bioavailability after subcutaneous injection, with an elimination half-life of 17 hours, allowing once-daily dosing. Due to its renal elimination, fondaparinux is contraindicated if the eGFR (estimated glomerular filtration rate) is <20 mL/min per $1.73\ m^2$.
- OASIS-5 – a randomised controlled trial in high-risk patients with unstable angina or MI without ST-segment elevation who received either fondaparinux, 2.5 mg daily or enoxaparin, 1 mg/kg of body weight twice daily – found fondaparinux to be non-inferior to enoxaparin in reducing the risk of ischaemic events, but substantially reduced major bleeding and improved long-term mortality and morbidity.[9]
- In patients pretreated with fondaparinux (2.5 mg subcutaneously once daily) undergoing percutaneous angioplasty, a single IV bolus of unfractionated heparin (70–85 IU/kg) is recommended during the procedure.
- In current ESC guidelines for management of acute coronary syndrome, fondaparinux (2.5 mg daily)

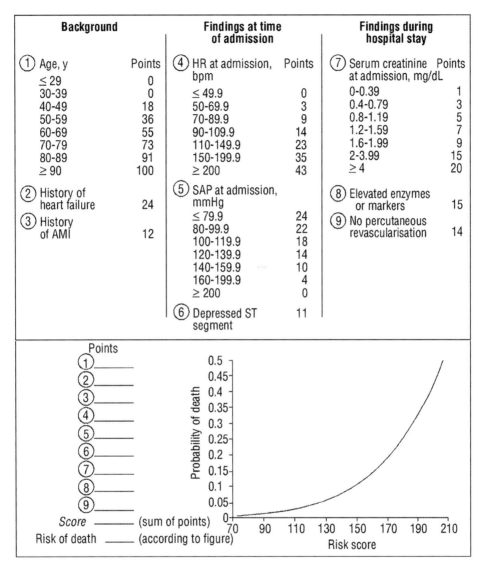

FIG. 5.4 The GRACE risk score. (Reproduced with permission from Fox KA, Fitzgerald G, Puymirat E, Huang W, Carruthers K, Simon T, et al. Should patients with acute coronary disease be stratified for management according to their risk? Derivation, external validation and outcomes using the updated GRACE risk score. *BMJ Open* 2014;4:e004425.)

is recommended as having the most favourable efficacy–safety profile regardless of the management strategy.[10]

Bivalirudin

- The direct thrombin inhibitor bivalirudin is administered intravenously. In the ACUITY trial,[11] patients diagnosed with NSTEMI and planned to treat in an invasive strategy were randomised into three treatment arms: UFH or LMWH with a GP IIb/IIIa receptor inhibitor, bivalirudin with a GP IIb/IIIa receptor inhibitor, or bivalirudin alone. Bivalirudin alone was found to be non-inferior to the standard UFH/LMWH combined with GP IIb/IIIa inhibitor, but there was a significantly lower rate of major bleeding with bivalirudin.

- The current CSANZ 2016 guideline[12] recommends considering bivalirudin (0.75 mg/kg IV with 1.75 mg/kg per hour infusion), as an alternative to glycoprotein IIb/IIIa inhibition and heparin, in patients with ACS undergoing angioplasty (PCI) with clinical features associated with an increased risk of bleeding events.[11]

Unfractionated Heparin

- UFH produces its major anticoagulant effect by inactivating thrombin and activated factor X (factor Xa) through an antithrombin (AT)-dependent mechanism.
- UFH has a narrow therapeutic window that requires monitoring. Its initial loading dose is 60 IU/kg IV (maximum 4000 IU), with an initial infusion of 12 IU/kg per hour (maximum 1000 IU/h), adjusted per activated partial thromboplastin time (aPTT) to maintain therapeutic anticoagulation (aPTT 1.5–2.5 × control) according to the specific hospital protocol, continued for 48 hours or until PCI is performed. UFH requires no dose adjustment in the presence of stage 5 chronic kidney disease.

Dawn had another episode of chest pain while in the emergency department. An ECG at the time of chest pain showed ST depression in LII, LIII and aVF. Her troponin was positive. She was transferred to the CCU and was treated with aspirin, ticagrelor, enoxaparin, atorvastatin and metoprolol.

Dawn was pain free for most of the day. The next day she had a coronary angiography that showed 90% narrowing of the RCA. She also had 50% narrowing of the LAD. Her left ventricular systolic function was normal.

Her right coronary artery was dilated and stented with a drug-eluting stent. She was advised to stop smoking and take on a healthy active life style. She was discharged home on day 3 with a follow-up appointment.

REFERENCES

1. Klinkman MS, Stevens D, Gorenflo DW. Episodes of care for chest pain: a preliminary report from MIRNET. *J Fam Pract* 1994;**38**:349.
2. Anderson JL, Adams CD, Antman EM, Bridges CR, Califf RM, Casey DE Jr, et al. ACCF/AHA focused update incorporated into the ACCF/AHA 2007 guidelines for the management of patients with unstable angina/non–ST elevation myocardial infarction: a report of the American College of Cardiology Foundation/American Heart Association Task Force on Practice Guidelines. *J Am Coll Cardiol* 2012;**61**(23):e179–347.
3. Chew DP, Scott IA, Cullen L, French JK, Briffa TG, Tideman PA, et al; NHFA/CSANZ ACS Guideline 2016 Executive Working Group. National Heart Foundation of Australia & Cardiac Society of Australia and New Zealand: Australian clinical guidelines for the management of acute coronary syndromes 2016. *Heart Lung Circ* 2016;**25**(9):895–951.
4. Thygesen K, Alpert JS, Jaffe AS, Simoons ML, Chaitman BR, White HD, ESC Committee for Practice Guidelines (CPG). Third universal definition of myocardial infarction. *Eur Heart J* 2012;**33**:2551–67.
5. Cullen L, Greenslade J, Merollini K, Graves N, Hammett CJ, Hawkins T, et al. Cost and outcomes of assessing patients with chest pain in an Australian emergency department. *Med J Aust* 2015;**202**(8):427–32.
6. Antman EM, Cohen MK, Bernink PJLM, McCabe CH, Horacek T, Papuchis G, et al. The TIMI risk score for unstable angina/non-ST elevation MI. *JAMA* 2000;**284**:835–42.
7. Fox KA, Fitzgerald G, Puymirat E, Huang W, Carruthers K, Simon T, et al. Should patients with acute coronary disease be stratified for management according to their risk? Derivation, external validation and outcomes using the updated GRACE risk score. *BMJ Open* 2014;**4**:e004425.
8. Granger CB, Goldberg RJ, Dabbous OH, Pieper KS, Eagle KA, Cannon CP, et al; the Global Registry of Acute Coronary Events Investigators. Predictors of hospital mortality in the global registry of acute coronary events. *Arch Intern Med* 2003;**163**:2345–53.
9. The Fifth Organization to Assess Strategies in Acute Ischemic Syndromes (OASIS-5) investigators and committees. *N Engl J Med* 2006;**354**:1464–76.
10. Roffi M, Patrono C, Collet JP, Mueller C, Valgimigli M, Andreotti F, et al. 2015 ESC Guidelines for the management of acute coronary syndromes in patients presenting without persistent ST-segment elevation. *Eur Heart J* 2016;**37**(3):267–315.
11. Stone GW, McLaurin BT, Cox DA, Bertrand ME, Lincoff AM, Moses JW, et al. Bivalirudin for patients with acute coronary syndromes. *N Engl J Med* 2006;**355**:2203–16.
12. National Heart Foundation of Australia & Cardiac Society of Australia and New Zealand: Australian clinical guidelines for the management of acute coronary syndromes 2016. *Heart Lung Circ* 2016;**25**:895–951.

Common Causes of ST Elevation in ECG[a]

CASE 8 SCENARIO: JULIA WITH CHEST PAIN AND ST ELEVATION

Julia, a 72-year-old previously well woman, felt lightheaded and experienced severe lower chest pain when at the shopping mall. She was taken to the nearest hospital within 45 minutes of the onset of pain. On arrival, her blood pressure was 180/103 mmHg and she looked pale. An ECG (Fig. 6.1) and troponin test were performed as part of her work-up.

Julia's history included hypertension and hypercholesterolaemia, and she is a lifelong smoker. She had no relevant family history and no previous cardiac events. She had recently travelled from another state to look after her daughter, who had had surgery.

Julia's ECG showed left ventricular hypertrophy (Box 6.1, Table 6.1).[1–4] She had borderline ST elevation (<2 mm) in lead VI and ST depression with T-wave inversion in LI, LII, LIII, aVF and V4–V6. A chest x-ray revealed a widened mediastinum and a CT aortogram showed large dissection of the thoracic aorta. Julia was immediately transferred to the nearest tertiary hospital while blood pressure-lowering treatment and adequate analgesia were continued. Fortunately, Julia did not receive any thrombolytic treatment, antiplatelet agents or heparin.

---

[a]Initially published as Atifur Rahman, Jilani Latona. Common causes of ST elevation. *Cardiology Today* 2017;7(1):29–34, reproduced with permission.

BOX 6.1
ECG Criteria for Diagnosing Left Ventricular Hypertrophy[1–4]

Many different ECG criteria for diagnosing left ventricular hypertrophy have been proposed over the years. Most use the voltage in one or more leads, with or without additional factors such as QRS duration, secondary ST–T wave abnormalities or left atrial abnormalities. The most well known electrocardiographic criteria are:

- Sokolow–Lyon criteria: S wave in VI plus the R wave in V5 or V6 is 35 mm.[1]
- Cornell criteria: R wave in aVL and the S wave in V3 is 28 mm in males or 20 mm in females.[2]
- Modified Cornell criteria: R wave in aVL is 12 mm.[3]
- Romhilt–Estes left ventricular hypertrophy point score system (see Table 6.1).[4]

ASSESSMENT OF CHEST PAIN

- Chest pain and other symptoms suggestive of acute coronary syndrome (ACS) are among the most common reasons for patients seeking medical attention. The underlying causes of such presentations may range from minor diseases such as musculoskeletal pain to life-threatening conditions such as acute myocardial infarction (AMI), aortic dissection or pulmonary embolism.

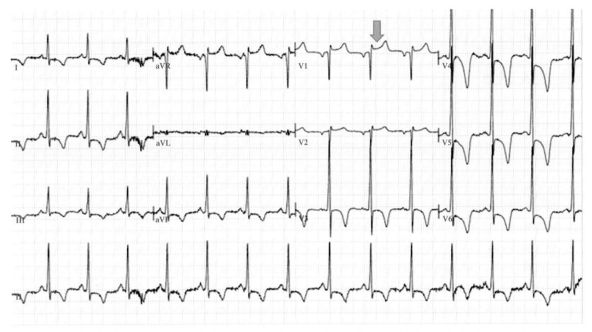

FIG. 6.1 High QRS voltage with diffuse T-wave inversion in a patient with left ventricular hypertrophy associated with ST elevation in lead V1 (arrow) and ST depression most obvious in leads V4 to V6.

TABLE 6.1
Romhilt–Estes LVH Point Score System[4]

Criteria	Points
VOLTAGE CRITERIA (ANY OF)	
R or S in limb leads ≥20 mm S wave in V1 or V2 ≥30 mm R wave in V5 or V6 ≥30 mm	3
ST–T ABNORMALITIES	
ST–T vector opposite to QRS without digitalis	3
ST–T vector opposite to QRS with digitalis	1
Normal ST–T vector	0
P-WAVE ABNORMALITIES	
Negative terminal P mode in V1 ≥1 mm in depth or 0.04 s in duration	3
OTHERS	
Left axis deviation (QRS of −30 degrees or more)	2
Delayed intrinsicoid deflection in V5 or V6 (>0.05 s)	1
QRS duration ≥0.09 s	1

Scoring system: 3 points or less=no signs of left ventricular hypertrophy; 4 points=probable left ventricular hypertrophy; 5 or more points=positive for left ventricular hypertrophy.

- Patients with chest pain require a prompt diagnosis. This can be achieved by taking a focused history, conducting a clinical examination and performing basic investigations including an ECG, a chest x-ray and blood tests. Failing to diagnose a life-threatening condition can result in mortality and serious morbidity for the patient and also represents a frequent cause of medical negligence cases.[5]

- A delayed diagnosis of MI can mean that a patient misses the window of opportunity for immediate thrombolysis or primary angioplasty. The ECG plays an important role in the early diagnosis of acute STEMI. It must be recorded before any reperfusion strategy can be initiated. Although ST elevation in a standard 12-lead ECG is an important factor to consider in the treatment of MI, several clinical conditions can result in ST elevation mimicking AMI (Table 6.2).

- In a US prospective observational study it was found that, in the emergency setting, ST-segment and T-wave abnormalities were frequently misread, with 41% false negatives and 14% false positives.[6] Although AMI needs to be considered first and foremost in the presence of ST elevation, it is not always the cause in clinical practice. A retrospective ECG review of adults with chest pain found only 15% of patients had STEMI and 85% of patients with ST elevation had a non-AMI diagnosis responsible for the ST elevation.[7] Thrombolysis in the wrong clinical setting

TABLE 6.2
Acute Myocardial Infarction and Other Conditions That Cause ST Elevation

Condition	Other ECG Features	Clinical Features
Acute myocardial infarction (AMI)	• ST elevation in one vascular territory • ST elevation with convex or straight pattern is traditionally considered as indicative of AMI in contrast to a concave pattern, which is typically considered to be secondary to non-ischaemic causes • Reciprocal ST depression in the opposite leads	• Typical or atypical chest pain or discomfort • Risk factors for coronary artery disease • Positive cardiac biomarkers
Left ventricular hypertrophy (LVH)	• High QRS voltage • ST and T-wave changes • (L) atrial enlargement • (L) axis deviation	• Patient may have history of hypertension, aortic regurgitation or stenosis or other valvular heart disease
Left bundle branch block (LBBB)	• Typically, ST and T waves are opposite in direction to the terminal QRS (appropriate discordance) • In myocardial infarction in the presence of previous LBBB, ST and T waves go to the same direction of the QRS complex (inappropriate concordance) • Extreme ST elevation in V1 and V2 leads may at times indicate ischaemia • QRS duration >0.12 seconds	• Commonly associated with hypertension, ischaemic heart disease and cardiomyopathy • Comparison with the old ECG is helpful
Pericarditis	• P–R interval depression • Diffuse ST-segment elevation with upward concavity • Reciprocal PR segment elevation (single arrows) and ST-segment depression (double arrows) in leads aVR and (occasionally) V1	• Characteristic clinical findings in pericarditis include pleuritic chest pain and a pericardial friction rub on auscultation • The most common aetiologies of pericarditis are idiopathic and viral
Hyperkalaemia	• ST elevation can be striking at times • Elevated ST segment often slopes down • Other ECG features of hyperkalaemia are often present including a wide QRS complex, tall, pointed, tented T wave and low-amplitude or absent P wave	• More common with increasing age in patients with diabetes and chronic kidney disease who are taking medications including ACE inhibitors, angiotensin receptor blockers, spironolactone or eplerenone
Early repolarisation	• Notch at the 'J' point (at the junction of ST segment and T wave) • Concave ST elevation • Most marked in V4 lead	• Absent cardiac biomarker elevation • Present in about 3% of healthy individuals
Takotsubo cardiomyopathy	• ST-segment elevation, most commonly in precordial leads • Diffuse deep symmetric T-wave inversion	• Classical patient is postmenopausal and presents with chest pain following an intense emotional or physical stress
Pulmonary embolism	• Sinus tachycardia • Complete or incomplete (R) bundle branch block • S1Q3T3 pattern • ST elevation or T-wave inversion in inferior or septal leads	• Typically the patient presents with dyspnoea, pleuritic chest pain, syncope following surgery or immobilisation

TABLE 6.2
Acute Myocardial Infarction and Other Conditions That Cause ST Elevation—cont'd

Condition	Other ECG Features	Clinical Features
Left ventricular aneurysm	• Persistent ST-segment elevation • Presence of Q waves	• May have a history of previous myocardial infarction
Normal ST elevation	• ST elevation in the precordial leads • The ST elevation is usually upwardly concave and is most marked in V2	• Common in younger men
Brugada syndrome	• Typical ECG findings include a right bundle branch block (RBBB) pattern • ST elevation in the right precordial leads (V1 and V3)	• Family history of Brugada syndrome or sudden cardiac death may be present
Coronary artery spasm	• Often dramatic, transient ST elevation.	• May present with early morning chest pain • May have history of substance abuse including cocaine and amphetamine use

can result in catastrophic complications such as fatal intracranial haemorrhage and death.

This chapter discusses common causes of ST elevation in the standard 12-lead ECG mimicking STEMI and the ways to differentiate these conditions.

ECG IN ACUTE MYOCARDIAL INFARCTION

- An ECG is considered to be an essential part of the diagnosis and evaluation of chest pain. Patients with typical ST elevation or new left bundle branch block are usually referred for immediate reperfusion therapy. An ECG in the setting of AMI can help localise the infarct, identify the coronary artery involved and predict the infarct size and prognosis.
- STEMI is typically confined to a single vascular territory and has an upwardly convex shape (Table 6.3).[8,9] Often there is reciprocal ST depression in the opposite leads (Fig. 6.2). In the early stages of AMI, the ECG may show a tall peaked T wave followed by ST elevation. As the condition progresses, the ECG shows Q-wave and T-wave inversion.
- In the current Australian guidelines, the ECG criteria for the diagnosis of STEMI are development of new left bundle branch block or persistent (>20 minutes) ST elevation in two or more leads[10]:
  - of 2.5 mm in leads V2 to V3 in men under 40 years
  - of 2 mm in V2 to V3 in men over 40 years
  - of 1.5 mm in V2 to V3 in women
  - of 1 mm or more ST elevation in other leads.

OTHER CAUSES OF ST ELEVATION

ECG Criteria for Diagnosing Left Ventricular Hypertrophy

- Left ventricular hypertrophy is frequently associated with secondary ST-segment or T-wave abnormalities. The ST segment and T wave are directed opposite to the QRS complex; this is called discordance between the QRS complex and the ST–T abnormalities. That means, typically, that there is ST elevation in the precordial leads, V1 and V2 (see Fig. 6.1) where the QRS complex is predominantly negative. In leads I, II, aVL, V4, V5 and V6, where the QRS complex is upright, the ST segment is often depressed (strain pattern).
- ST elevation due to LVH is typically concave, and other features of LVH (see Table 6.1, Box 6.1) are present.[1-4] In a retrospective review of the ECGs from adults with chest pain presenting to an emergency department, LVH was found most often to be responsible (25%) for electrocardiographic ST elevation.[7]

ST Elevation in Takotsubo Cardiomyopathy

- Takotsubo cardiomyopathy mimics AMI in presentation and should be considered in all postmenopausal women who present with chest pain after intense emotional or physical stress; however, in 20%–35% of cases there is no obvious precipitant. The patient may also present with dyspnoea, palpitations, syncope, cardiac arrest or ECG changes. Although a chest x-ray may be normal, the patient may present with acute pulmonary oedema and cardiomegaly.

Location	Artery Involved	ECG Features
TABLE 6.3 Localisation of Infarct, Artery Involved and ECG Findings in Patients With Acute Myocardial Infarction[8,9]		
Inferior	Right coronary artery (RCA) Left circumflex (L Cx)	Greater ST elevation in LIII compared with LII ST depression in LI and aVL Isoelectric or elevated ST segment in LI, aVL, V5 and V6 (in addition to ST elevation in LII, LIII and aVF)
Right ventricle infarction	Proximal RCA	ST elevation in V4R (right-sided chest lead) ST elevation in V1 associated with ST elevation in II, III and aVF
Posterior	Posterior descending artery – usually a branch of the RCA	ECG changes are mirror image of an anteroseptal MI: • R/S ratio in V1 or V2 >1 • Hyperacute ST–T-wave changes: i.e. ST depression and large, inverted T waves in V1 to V3 Posterior infarction is confirmed by the presence of ST elevation and Q waves in the posterior leads (V7 to V9)
Anterior	Left anterior descending artery (LAD) Proximal LAD Distal LAD	Anterior=V2 to V5 Anteroseptal=V1 to V3 Extensive anterior=V1 to V6, I and aVL Prominent ST elevation in I and aVL and inferior ST depression is consistent with proximal LAD occlusion ST depression in aVL particularly if combined with isoelectric ST segments in the inferior leads suggests distal LAD occlusion
Lateral	• Diagonal branch of the LAD • Obtuse marginal branch of (L)Cx • Ramus intermedius	ST elevation in the lateral leads (LI, aVL, V5 and V6) Reciprocal ST depression in the inferior leads (III and aVF)

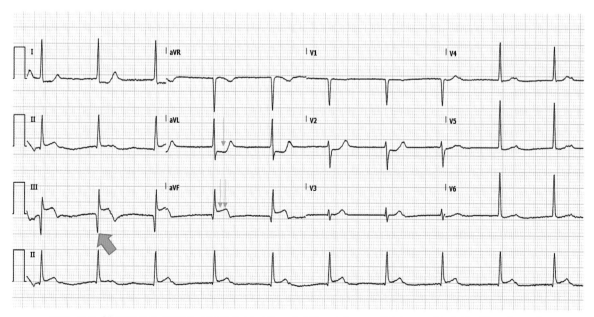

FIG. 6.2 ST elevation (double arrow) in LII, LIII and aVF and Q wave (thick arrow) in L III with reciprocal ST depression (single arrow) in a patient with acute inferior myocardial infarction.

- The most common acute ECG findings of takotsubo cardiomyopathy are ST elevation in the precordial leads and T-wave inversion in almost all leads.[11] Unlike the situation in AMI, the ECG changes in takotsubo cardiomyopathy are not limited to one vascular territory. ECG findings are often dramatic and not in proportion with the changes in the patient's troponin levels. Patients also may develop pathological Q waves that typically resolve before hospital discharge, with restoration of normal R-wave progression, There may also be a prolonged Q–T interval (beginning of Q wave to end of T wave) which usually normalises in 1 to 2 days, or a prolonged P–R interval (beginning of the P wave to beginning of the QRS complex).[12]
- The diffuse ST elevation that does not follow any particular vascular territory and the absence of reciprocal ST changes make the diagnosis of STEMI unlikely. ST elevation in patients with myocardial infarction is often associated with reciprocal changes in leads III and aVL.

ST Elevation in Pericarditis

- In patients with acute pericarditis, the ST segment is elevated diffusely, with upward concavity in the precordial and the limb leads (Fig. 6.3A). The ST elevation usually involves more than one coronary vascular territory and there is an absence of reciprocal ST changes in leads III and aVL. In patients with pericarditis the PR segment is depressed, but this is not specific for acute pericarditis as early repolarisation or atrial infarction can also cause the depression.[13,14] In lead aVR, and occasionally in lead V1, there may be a reciprocal PR segment elevation and ST-segment depression (Fig. 6.3B).
- Acute myocarditis can cause diffuse ST elevation similar to that seen in pericarditis. In this case, the absence of any systemic symptoms and absence of a prior illness make the diagnosis of pericarditis or myocarditis unlikely.

ST Elevation in Early Repolarisation

- Early repolarisation is characterised by ST elevation with a concave morphology (Fig. 6.3C) and notching of the J point (the junction where the QRS complex ends and the ST segment begins). It is seen in leads with a tall R wave and is most marked in V4 (V2 to V5). Rarely, it can involve the inferior leads. It occurs in 2%–5% of the population, predominantly in young males. Reciprocal changes classically seen in patients with AMI are generally absent. Unless the patient is having an acute coronary syndrome, the cardiac biomarker troponin should be negative.

- Although it is sometimes called 'benign early repolarisation', whether it is a totally benign condition or carries a slightly increased risk of sudden cardiac death remains controversial. A Finnish study found that patients with J-point elevation of more than 0.1 mV in the inferior or lateral leads were about 1.3 times more likely to die from sudden cardiac death, whereas those who had J-point elevation of more than 0.2 mV were three times more likely to have sudden cardiac death.[15] On the other hand, no significant association between any components of early repolarisation and cardiac mortality have been found.[16]

Normal Variant ST Elevation

- A study of 6014 asymptomatic men, conducted to help define the normal ECG and to delineate the range of variation, found that ST elevation in the precordial leads is very common (91.2%). ST elevation was most marked (Fig. 6.3D) in the anterior leads (elevation in V2 to V4; 43.8%), followed by the lateral leads (elevation in V3 to V6; 24%), anterolateral leads (elevation in all precordial leads; 16.8%) and rightward (elevation in V1 to V2 only; 6.8%). Only 8.8% of men had no ST elevation in any precordial leads, 44.3% had 0.1 mV ST elevation, 38.4% had 0.2 mV ST elevation and 0.1% had ST elevation of 0.5 mV. The ST elevation is usually upwardly concave and is most marked in V2. ST elevation is common in younger men and the prevalence decreases with age.[17]

ST Elevation in Left Bundle Branch Block (LBBB)

- The guidelines for the management of patients with AMI recommend immediate revascularisation with thrombolysis or primary angioplasty for patients with chest pain and new LBBB.[10] ECG changes in the presence of preexisting LBBB are slightly more complex because ST-segment and T-wave changes including ST elevation and ST depression in the presence of LBBB are common.[10]
- Normally in LBBB, the ST segments and T waves are opposite in direction to the terminal QRS deflection (Fig. 6.3E). These changes are secondary to the bundle branch block itself (secondary ST-segment and T-wave changes). This means that in the presence of LBBB the septal leads (V1 to V3) quite often show ST elevation and an upright T wave where the QRS complex is predominantly negative. There is also association with ST depression and T-wave inversion in the lateral leads (V5 and V6) where the QRS complex

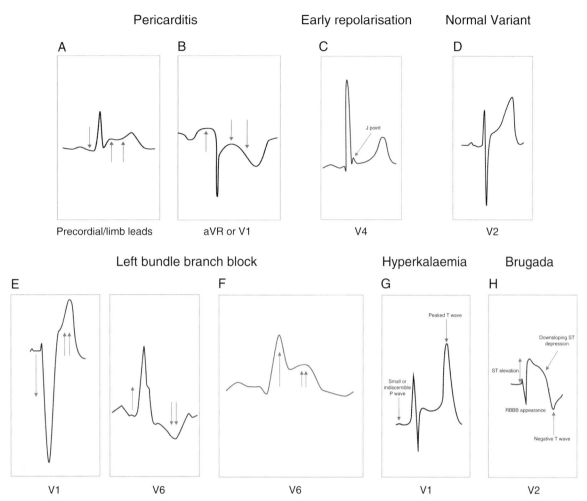

FIG. 6.3 **(A)** Pericarditis showing diffuse ST-segment elevation (double arrow) and PR depression (single arrow), and **(B)** reciprocal PR-segment elevation (single arrow) and ST-segment depression (double arrow) in a VR and occasionally in V1. **(C)** Early repolarisation: ST elevation with a concave morphology and notching of the J point. **(D)** Normal variant: ST elevation in precordial leads in younger men. Left bundle branch block (LBBB): **(E)** the QRS complexes (single arrow) and the ST segment (double arrow) go in opposite directions (appropriate discordance) secondary to intraventricular conduction delay, and **(F)** the QRS complex (single arrow) and the ST segment (double arrow) go in the same directions (inappropriate concordance), suggestive of ischaemia. **(G)** Hyperkalaemia. **(H)** Brugada syndrome.

is predominantly positive. This is called 'appropriate discordance'.

- ST elevation in association with a positive QRS complex (in V4 to V6) or ST depression in leads that have predominantly negative QRS complexes (V1 to V3) is not expected in patients with uncomplicated LBBB and is termed 'inappropriate concordance' (Fig. 6.3F). It strongly indicates the presence of acute ischaemia.

- In patients with LBBB, the modified Sgarbossa criteria are useful in identifying STEMI: ST elevation of more than 1 mm concordant with QRS (five points), ST depression of more than 1 mm in leads V1 to V3 (three points) and ST elevation more than 5 mm discordant with QRS (two points).[10,18] A score of more than three points is associated with 98% chance of having MI, but a score of 0 does not rule out STEMI.

ECG Features of Hyperkalaemia

- ST elevation in hyperkalaemia can be striking at times (Fig. 6.3G).[19] Other ECG features of hyperkalaemia that can be present are widened QRS complexes, tall, pointed T waves and low-amplitude or absent P waves. In hyperkalaemia the ST segment is often downward sloping.
- Hyperkalaemia is more common with increasing age and in patients with diabetes and chronic kidney disease who take medications that block the renin–angiotensin–aldosterone system including ACE inhibitors, angiotensin receptor blockers, direct renin inhibitors and aldosterone receptor antagonists such as spironolactone or eplerenone.

ECG Features of Left Ventricular Aneurysm

- A left ventricular aneurysm can be diagnosed on the ECG when there is persistent ST-elevation-associated Q waves after a transmural myocardial infarction. In a patient with an anterior or apical aneurysm, the persistent ST elevation is most marked in leads V1 and V2. In a patient with an aneurysm after an inferior MI, changes are marked in LII, LIII and aVF.[20]
- The patient's history of a previous infarct and an echocardiography are helpful in documenting the presence of an aneurysm. The shape of the ST elevation is also relatively specific and has been described as 'coving' (over Q waves).

ECG Features of Brugada Syndrome

- Brugada syndrome is a familial disease with an autosomal dominant mode of transmission. The family history is often positive for sudden cardiac death at a young age, most commonly occurring during sleep and in particular during the early morning hours.[21]
- Typical ECG findings in Brugada syndrome include a right bundle branch block (RBBB) pattern and ST elevation in the right precordial leads (V1 and V3) in the absence of long Q–T intervals and any structural disease (Fig. 6.3H).[22] The ST elevation can have a saddleback shape, but in typical cases the ST segment is downward sloping and ends with an inverted T wave. ST elevation in Brugada syndrome may be present intermittently. Challenging the patient with a sodium channel blocker such as flecainide can unmask a typical electrocardiographic pattern.[23]

ECG Features of Pulmonary Embolism

- The ECG features of pulmonary embolism include sinus tachycardia, simultaneous T-wave inversion in the inferior (II, III and aVF) and right precordial (V1 to V4) leads, ST elevation, S1Q3T3 pattern (deep S wave in lead I, Q wave in III, inverted T wave in III) and complete or incomplete RBBB. ST elevation in the presence of massive pulmonary embolism can be striking at times.[24]
- Consider pulmonary embolism as a differential diagnosis in any patient who presents with pleuritic chest pain, dyspnoea or syncope in the postoperative setting, after prolonged immobilisation. Patients with malignancy or inherited blood-clotting disorders are also at increased risk. Patients may have an elevated jugular venous pressure and other signs of right ventricular cardiac failure. A D-dimer test is very helpful in excluding pulmonary embolism as it is considered a highly sensitive test for pulmonary embolism and a negative test makes diagnosis of pulmonary embolism unlikely. Unfortunately, D-dimer lacks specificity and has low positive predictive value. When clinical suspicion of pulmonary embolism is high, a CT pulmonary angiogram may be needed to confirm the diagnosis.

ST Elevation in Coronary Artery Spasm

- Spasm of an epicardial coronary artery can produce dramatic, transient ST elevation in patients with chest pain. Although coronary spasm is usually brief and the ST segment returns to normal without myocardial injury, prolonged spasm can result in myocardial infarction.[25] Withdrawal vagal tone is most often the mechanism leading to spontaneous spasm.
- Patients with coronary artery spasm are usually younger than those who present with unstable angina or chronic stable angina and tend to present with early-morning chest pain. An important associated risk factor is substance abuse including tobacco and marijuana smoking, alcohol consumption and cocaine and amphetamine use.

CONCLUSION

The 12-lead ECG is an integral part of the diagnostic work-up of a patient with acute chest pain. It is the recommended bedside test to confirm or exclude the diagnosis of STEMI and, in the presence of ST elevation, myocardial infarction needs to be considered first and foremost.

ST elevation caused by conditions other than acute ischaemia is common. At times, distinguishing between STEMI from non-ischaemic causes of elevation of the ST segment is difficult, especially in patients with atypical presenting symptoms. Understanding of common patterns of ST elevation that are not caused by ischaemia is crucial for rapid and accurate diagnosis of STEMI and subsequent reperfusion strategy.

In certain clinical contexts, when equivocal ECG abnormalities are detected, other differential diagnoses should be considered in order to avoid unnecessary, potentially dangerous therapies. The use of serial ECGs, comparison with old ECGs and looking for ST elevation confined to single vascular territories with or without reciprocal ST depression can help with discrimination. Sometimes, obtaining expert help and, if it is available, remote ECG review can assist in the diagnosis of STEMI.

REFERENCES

1. Sokolow M, Lyon TP. The ventricular complex in left ventricular hypertrophy as obtained by unipolar precordial and limb leads. *Am Heart J* 1949;**37**:161–86.
2. Casale PN, Devereux RB, Kligfield P, Eisenberg RR, Miller DH, Chaudhary BS, et al. Electrocardiographic detection of left ventricular hypertrophy: development and prospective validation of improved criteria. *J Am Coll Cardiol* 1985;**6**:572–80.
3. Molloy TJ, Okin PM, Devereux RB, Kligfield P. Electrocardiographic detection of left ventricular hypertrophy by the simple QRS voltage-duration product. *J Am Coll Cardiol* 1992;**20**:1180–6.
4. Romhilt DW, Estes EH Jr. A point-score system for the ECG diagnosis of left ventricular hypertrophy. *Am Heart J* 1968;**75**:752–8.
5. Rusnak RA, Stair TO, Hansen K, Fastow JS. Litigation against the emergency physician: common features in cases of missed myocardial infarction. *Ann Emerg Med* 1989;**18**:1029–34.
6. Jayes RL, Larsen GC, Beshansky JR, D'Agostino RB, Selker HP. Physician electrocardiogram reading in the emergency department – accuracy and effect on triage decisions: findings from a multicenter study. *J Gen Intern Med* 1992;**7**:387–92.
7. Brady WJ, Perron AD, Martin ML, Beagle C, Aufderheide TP. Cause of ST segment abnormality in ED chest pain patients. *Am J Emerg Med* 2001;**19**:25–8.
8. Zimetbaum PJ, Josephson ME. Use of the electrocardiogram in acute myocardial infarction. *N Engl J Med* 2003;**348**:933–40.
9. Arbane M, Goy JJ. Prediction of the site of total occlusion in the left anterior descending coronary artery using admission electrocardiogram in anterior wall acute myocardial infarction. *Am J Cardiol* 2000;**85**:487–91.
10. Chew DP, Scott IA, Cullen L, French JK, Briffa TG, Tideman PA, et al; NHFA/CSANZ ACS Guideline 2016 Executive Working Group. National Heart Foundation of Australia &
Cardiac Society of Australia and New Zealand: Australian clinical guidelines for the management of acute coronary syndromes 2016. *Heart Lung Circ* 2016;**25**:895–951.
11. Rahman A, Liu D. Broken heart syndrome: a case study. *Aust Fam Physician* 2012;**41**(1/2):55–8.
12. Bybee KA, Kara T, Prasad A, Lerman A, Barsness GW, Wright RS, et al. Systematic review: transient left ventricular apical ballooning: a syndrome that mimics ST-segment elevation myocardial infarction. *Ann Intern Med* 2004;**141**:858–65.
13. Spodick DH. Diagnostic electrocardiographic sequences in acute pericarditis: significance of PR segment and PR vector changes. *Circulation* 1973;**48**:575–80.
14. Rahman A, Liu D. Pericarditis: clinical features and management. *Aust Fam Physician* 2011;**40**:791–6.
15. Tikkanen JT, Anttonen O, Junttila MJ, Aro AL, Kerola T, Rissanen HA, et al. Long-term outcome associated with early repolarization on electrocardiography. *N Engl J Med* 2009;**361**:2529–37.
16. Uberoi A, Jain NA, Perez M, Weinkopff A, Ashley E, Hadley D, et al. Early repolarization in an ambulatory clinical population. *Circulation* 2011;**124**:2208–14.
17. Hiss RG, Lamb LE, Allen MF. Electrocardiographic findings in 67,375 asymptomatic subjects. *Am J Cardiol* 1960;**6**:200–31.
18. Sgarbossa EB, Pinski SL, Barbagelata A, Underwood DA, Gates KB, Topol EJ. Electrocardiographic diagnosis of evolving acute myocardial infarction in the presence of left bundle-branch block. *N Engl J Med* 1996;**334**:481–7.
19. Sims DB, Sperling LS. Images in cardiovascular medicine. ST-segment elevation resulting from hyperkalemia. *Circulation* 2005;**111**:e295–6.
20. Smith SW. T/QRS ratio best distinguishes ventricular aneurysm from anterior myocardial infarction. *Am J Emerg Med* 2005;**23**:279–87.
21. Matsuo K, Kurita T, Inagaki M, Kakishita M, Aihara N, Shimizu W, et al. The circadian pattern of the development of ventricular fibrillation in patients with Brugada syndrome. *Eur Heart J* 1999;**20**:465–70.
22. Brugada P, Brugada J. Right bundle branch block, persistent ST segment elevation and sudden cardiac death: a distinct clinical and electrocardiographic syndrome: a multicenter report. *J Am Coll Cardiol* 1992;**20**:1391–6.
23. Brugada R, Brugada J, Antzelevitch C, Kirsch GE, Potenza D, Towbin JA, et al. Sodium channel blockers identify risk for sudden death in patients with ST-segment elevation and right bundle branch block but structurally normal hearts. *Circulation* 2000;**101**:510–15.
24. Wang K, Asinger RW, Marriott HJ. ST-segment elevation in conditions other than acute myocardial infarction. *N Engl J Med* 2003;**349**:2128–35.
25. Stern S, Bayes de Luna A. Coronary artery spasm: a 2009 update. *Circulation* 2009;**119**:2531–4.

CHAPTER 7

Coronary Artery Disease

KEY POINTS

- Stable coronary artery disease is generally characterised by a reversible mismatch between myocardial demand and supply, usually due to epicardial coronary artery stenosis.
- In-stent restenosis (ISR) is caused by neointimal hyperplasia. ISR may be associated with a recurrence of stable angina symptoms in most patients.
- Coronary stent thrombosis is a serious and potentially life-threatening complication after coronary stenting. It is more likely to cause an acute coronary syndrome than stable angina.
- The exercise stress test (EST) is a functional test that is useful in assessment and risk stratification of chest pain in patients with intermediate probability for coronary artery disease. It is a simple, widely available and cost-effective technique.
- A stress echocardiogram, which combines a standard EST with an echocardiogram taken before and immediately after exercise, gives higher specificity for detecting coronary artery disease. Compared with nuclear imaging, stress echocardiography has similar accuracy and markedly higher specificity.
- A myocardial perfusion scan with dipyridamole is indicated for assessing chest pain in patients who are unable to exercise adequately or have an abnormal baseline ECG (e.g. left bundle branch block (LBBB)).
- A CT coronary angiogram provides additional information non-invasively about the vessel condition, remodelling and plaque surrounding the lumen.
- Coronary angiography is an invasive procedure which remains the 'gold standard' in detecting coronary artery disease and luminal narrowing.

CASE 9 SCENARIO: DAWN WITH NON-ST ELEVATION MYOCARDIAL INFARCTION

Dawn remained well for 6 months after her recent non-ST elevation myocardial infarction and stent to the (R) coronary artery. She had residual 50% non-obstructive stenosis of her left anterior descending artery noted on her initial angiogram.

She has been active and stopped smoking after the heart attack. She has been well and taking medications, including dual antiplatelet agents regularly. Last week, when mowing her lawn, she felt a brief episode of chest pain which was quickly relieved by sublingual nitrate treatment.

Question

True statements about Dawn's condition may include:
1. *Dawn may have developed 'in-stent restenosis'.*
2. *Her presentation is unlikely to be due to 'stent thrombosis'.*
3. *If she is symptomatic despite optimum medical treatment, she may require further tests.*
4. *Initial investigations to diagnose her symptoms should include a resting ECG.*

PATHOGENESIS OF ANGINA PECTORIS IN STABLE CORONARY ARTERY DISEASE

- Angina in stable coronary artery disease is generally characterised by reversible mismatch between myocardial demand and supply, due to ischaemia. Symptoms are usually induced by exercise (increased demand) and relieved by rest.
- The likely causes are: epicardial coronary artery stenosis, microvascular dysfunction, vasoconstriction or a combination of these.[1]

Stent Failure: Stent Thrombosis vs Restenosis

The two major causes of stent failure are stent thrombosis and in-stent restenosis (ISR). Improved procedural techniques and the widespread use of new-generation drug-eluting stents (DESs) have dramatically reduced the incidence of both stent thrombosis and ISR.

In-Stent Restenosis

- Neointimal hyperplasia which is the cause of in-stent restenosis (Fig. 7.1; part A shows a normal

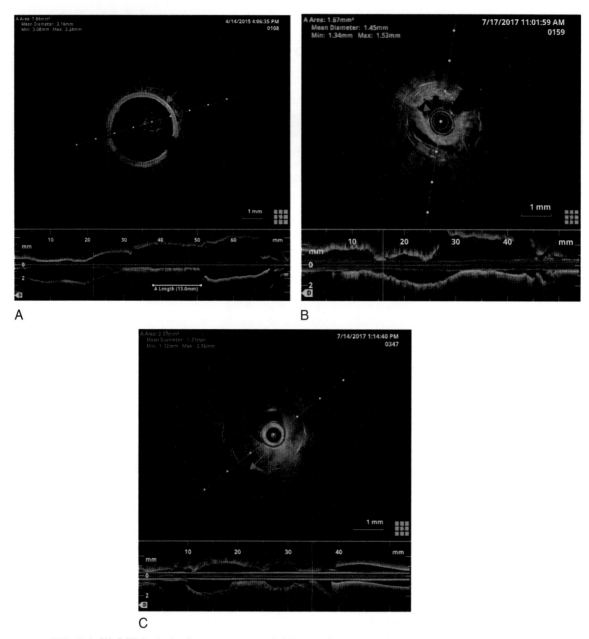

FIG. 7.1 **(A)** OCT (optical coherence tomography) image of a normal trilaminar coronary artery with outer adventitia, middle media (arrow showing dark circular line in between) and inner intima. **(B)** Thrombus (red arrow) in the previously stented right coronary artery. **(C)** In-stent restenosis due to homogeneous neointimal proliferation (double arrow); single arrow indicates previous stent struts.

artery, Fig. 7.1C shows in-stent restenosis) remains an obstacle to the long-term efficacy of stents. In general, the inflammatory response to vessel wall injury during angioplasty plays a central role in ISR after stenting, with vessel wall inflammation driving fibroblast growth and smooth muscle cell hyperplasia.[2]

- Angiographic follow-up has shown that neointimal hyperplasia results in in-stent restenosis in 20%–30% of cases after intervention with a BMS (bare-metal stent). With contemporary stents (DES), clinically relevant restenosis occurs in <5% cases at 12 months. ISR is associated with a recurrence of symptoms of stable angina in most patients.
- Angiographic surveillance studies have shown that neointimal hyperplasia after bare metal stenting tends to peak at 6 months after stenting and thereafter remain stable.
- Drug-eluting stents were introduced because of the frequency of ISR and the need for re-intervention in many of these patients. The release of an antiproliferative drug from the stent reduces neointimal proliferation and has dramatically reduced the need for re-intervention.

Stent Thrombosis

- Coronary stent thrombosis (Fig. 7.1B showing stent thrombosis, Fig. 7.1A showing a normal artery) is a serious and potentially life-threatening complication of coronary stenting. The true effect and incidence of stent thrombosis is uncertain. Stent thrombosis is, however, often a dramatic event, typically resulting in ST elevation myocardial infarction with high mortality rate.[3]
- Risk factors associated with stent thrombosis can be categorised as clinical-, angiographic- and procedure-related risk factors.
- Non-adherence and non-responsiveness to the prescribed dual antiplatelet therapy are factors that also play a major role.
- Problems with bleeding or the need for a surgical operation are quite common causes of cessation of antiplatelet treatment. It is important to remember that heparin is not effective as an alternative to antiplatelet drugs for these patients.

Predictors of Stent Thrombosis

These include the following:

- Procedural – e.g. undersizing of the stent, bifurcation stenting and dissection. This generally results in early (within the first 30 days) stent thrombosis.

- Clinical – e.g. diabetes, chronic kidney disease, young age, smoking, present malignancy and stenting for myocardial infarction (primary angioplasty).
- Angiographic – e.g. small vessel diameter, long stent and multivessel disease.
- In the Bern–Rotterdam registry, definite stent thrombosis occurred in 192 out of the 8146 patients (treated with either a sirolimus-eluting stent ($n=3823$) or a paclitaxel-eluting stent ($n=4323$)), with an incidence of $1/100$ patient-years and a cumulative incidence of 3.3% at 4 years.[4]
- The reported incidence of late (after 30 days) and very late stent thrombosis (after 360 days) in second-generation DESs, such as zotarolimus-eluting and everolimus-eluting stents., is very low.
- Recent results from a registry of 18,334 patients showed that the cumulative incidence of definite stent thrombosis at 3 years was 1.5% with BMS, 2.2% with first-generation DESs, and 1.0% with second-generation DESs.[5]

Six months after angioplasty, Dawn continued to have recurrent grade I chest pain with strenuous activity. She didn't have symptoms on ordinary physical activity or at rest (Table 7.1). Her chest pain is very typical of angina. The timing and pattern of her symptoms is highly suggestive of in-stent restenosis.

She had 50% non-obstructive coronary artery disease in her LAD that may also have progressed causing symptom. Late stent thrombosis after 6 months is less likely when she is taking dual antiplatelet agents regularly. Stent thrombosis generally does not cause stable coronary artery disease symptoms; rather it produces acute ST elevation myocardial infarction with a high mortality.

Dawn's antianginal drug, metoprolol, dosage was increased to 50 mg twice daily (Table 7.2). She was also prescribed a long-acting nitrate and it was arranged for her to have exercise stress echocardiography.

Other tests may be appropriate in Dawn's management.

INVESTIGATING CORONARY ARTERY DISEASE
Biochemical Tests

- Metabolic abnormalities – e.g. fasting blood glucose, HbA_{1c} – should be investigated as part of the evaluation of patients with angina.
- Thyroid function tests to assess for thyrotoxicosis (increased metabolic demands on the heart may cause angina).

TABLE 7.1
Canadian Cardiovascular Society Grading of Angina Pectoris

Grade	Description
Grade I	Ordinary physical activity does not cause angina, such as walking and climbing stairs. Angina with strenuous or rapid or prolonged exertion at work or recreation
Grade II	Slight limitation of ordinary activity. Walking or climbing stairs rapidly, walking uphill, walking or stair climbing after meals, or in cold, or in wind, or under emotional stress, or only during the few hours after awakening. Walking more than two blocks on the level and climbing more than one flight of ordinary stairs at a normal pace and in normal conditions
Grade III	Marked limitation of ordinary physical activity. Walking one or two blocks on the level and climbing one flight of stairs in normal conditions and at normal pace
Grade IV	Inability to carry on any physical activity without discomfort; angina may be present at rest

(Reference: Campeau L. Grading of angina pectoris. *Circulation* 1976;54:5223. Available on the Canadian Cardiovascular Society website at www.ccs.ca.)

- Evaluation for anaemia as a contributor of angina pain (not uncommon in patients taking dual antiplatelet drugs from occult gastrointestinal bleeding).
- Fasting lipid profile.

Resting ECG
- All patients with suspected angina should have a resting ECG.
- A normal ECG does not exclude the diagnosis of ischaemia.
- The resting ECG may show signs of previous myocardial infarction.

Non-Invasive Tests
The choice of the initial test should be based on the patient's resting ECG, physical ability to exercise, local expertise, and available technologies. The diagnosis of stable coronary artery disease may also be supported by functional testing (exercise ECG or an imaging stress test). Functional tests give additional important information about the causal relationship between ischaemia and the occurrence of the patient's symptoms.[1]

Exercise stress test[6]
- The exercise stress test (EST) is an important diagnostic and prognostic tool for assessing patients with a wide range of cardiac conditions. The test also provides additional information, such as workload achieved, heart rate response, blood pressure response and symptoms reproduced, which has both diagnostic and prognostic relevance.
- EST is a simple, widely available and low-cost technique. The usefulness of the EST depends on patient selection and pretest probability. Generally, standard EST has low sensitivity (relatively high false negative) but relatively high specificity (low false positive). EST has a sensitivity of 45% and a specificity of 85% for detecting coronary artery disease.
- False-positive results are more frequent in patients with an abnormal resting ECG, including left ventricular hypertrophy and those who use digoxin or have an intraventricular conduction defect or atrial fibrillation.
- Currently, EST is the most commonly used initial non-invasive test for diagnosing coronary artery disease.

Indications for exercise stress testing
- Assessment of chest pain in patients with intermediate probability for coronary artery disease (CAD).
- Assessment of functional capacity and prognosis of patients with known CAD.
- Evaluation of exercise-induced arrhythmias (patients who notice palpitations during exercise).
- Assessment of functional capacity and symptomatic responses in patients with a history of valvular heart disease and with equivocal symptoms.
- Assessment of cardiopulmonary function in patients with heart failure or pulmonary hypertension.
- EST should not be used to screen very-low-risk, asymptomatic individuals because the test has limited diagnostic and prognostic value in this situation.

Interpretation of EST
The main diagnostic ECG abnormality during ECG exercise testing consists of a horizontal or down-sloping ST-segment depression ≥1 mm, after the J point, in one or more ECG leads (Fig. 7.2).

Markers of adverse prognosis in EST
- Early onset of typical chest pain.
- No increase or a fall in systolic blood pressure during exercise.
- Horizontal or down-sloping ST segment depression >2 mm.

TABLE 7.2
Commonly Used Antianginal Drugs

Class	Common Drugs	Cautions	Notes
Beta-blockers	Metoprolol, atenolol, bisoprolol, carvedilol, nebivolol	Asthma, severe bradycardia, peripheral vascular disease, severe depression	First-line treatment for stable angina
Non-dihydropyridine CCBs	Verapamil, diltiazem	Bradyarrhythmias; heart failure with reduced systolic function; best avoided in combination with BBs	First-line treatment; controls heart rate and symptoms of angina; useful in vasospastic angina
Dihydropyridine CCBs	Nifedipine, amlodipine	Severe aortic stenosis, hypertrophic cardiomyopathy	Can be used with BBs; may increase heart rate
Sinus node (*f* channel) blocker	Ivabradine	Can cause bradycardia	Useful second-line agent in patients with sinus rhythm who cannot take BBs
Long-acting nitrate	Isosorbide di-nitrate, mononitrates	Headache is common, contraindicated in hypertrophic cardiomyopathy	Nitrate tolerance is common problem
Nitrate derivative	Nicorandil	Headache	Second-line drug after BBs, CCBs
Other agents	Perhexiline	Can precipitate severe hepatotoxicity or peripheral neuropathy; toxicity closely associated with plasma concentration >600 ng/mL	Monitoring of plasma; perhexiline concentration needed; levels must be elevated for at least 3 months to precipitate toxicity (honeymoon period)

BB = beta-blocker; CCB = calcium channel blocker.

- ST-segment elevation.
- Significant arrhythmias.

Stress echocardiography[7]
- The combination of echocardiography with a physical or pharmacological stress allows detection of myocardial ischaemia. A transient worsening of regional function during stress is the hallmark of inducible ischaemia.
- Pharmacological testing is preferred if the patient is unable to exercise adequately.
- It is the preferred non-invasive imaging technique owing to its low cost, wide availability and the lack of radiation exposure involved.
- Exercise, dobutamine and dipyridamole are the most frequently used stressors for stress echocardiography.
- In a meta-analysis of 55 studies with 3714 patients, exercise, dobutamine and dipyridamole echocardiography showed a sensitivity of 83%, 81% and 72% respectively, and a specificity of 84%, 84% and 95%.[8]

- The use of contrast during stress echocardiography enhances image quality; it also enhances its accuracy for the detection of coronary artery disease.

Myocardial perfusion scintigraphy using SPECT
Technetium -99m is the most commonly used of nuclear tracers and is now employed with single photon emission computed tomography (SPECT) in association with a symptom-limited exercise test. The sensitivity and specificity of exercise stress SPECT are 73%–92% and 63%–87% respectively. Thallium-201 is associated with a higher radiation than technetium and CT coronary angiography now involves considerably less radiation than either of them.[1,8]
- It is used to detect myocardial ischaemia.
- Tracer is taken up by healthy myocardium. The initial uptake, or extraction into cardiac myocytes, is directly proportional to regional blood flow.
- Ischaemia produces a 'cold' spot. Reduced regional trace uptake during stress compared with preserved

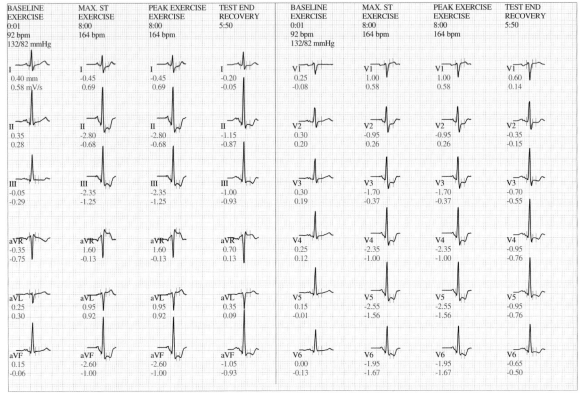

BASELINE EXERCISE 0:01 92 bpm 132/82 mmHg	MAX. ST EXERCISE 8:00 164 bpm	PEAK EXERCISE EXERCISE 8:00 164 bpm	TEST END RECOVERY 5:50	BASELINE EXERCISE 0:01 92 bpm 132/82 mmHg	MAX. ST EXERCISE 8:00 164 bpm	PEAK EXERCISE EXERCISE 8:00 164 bpm	TEST END RECOVERY 5:50
I 0.40 mm 0.58 mV/s	I -0.45 0.69	I -0.45 0.69	I -0.20 -0.05	V1 0.25 -0.08	V1 1.00 0.58	V1 1.00 0.58	V1 0.60 0.14
II 0.35 0.28	II -2.80 -0.68	II -2.80 -0.68	II -1.15 -0.87	V2 0.30 0.20	V2 -0.95 0.26	V2 -0.95 0.26	V2 -0.35 -0.15
III -0.05 -0.29	III -2.35 -1.25	III -2.35 -1.25	III -1.00 -0.93	V3 0.30 0.19	V3 -1.70 -0.37	V3 -1.70 -0.37	V3 -0.70 -0.55
aVR -0.35 -0.75	aVR 1.60 -0.13	aVR 1.60 -0.13	aVR 0.70 0.13	V4 0.25 0.12	V4 -2.35 -1.00	V4 -2.35 -1.00	V4 -0.95 -0.76
aVL 0.25 0.30	aVL 0.95 0.92	aVL 0.95 0.92	aVL 0.35 0.09	V5 0.15 -0.01	V5 -2.55 -1.56	V5 -2.55 -1.56	V5 -0.95 -0.76
aVF 0.15 -0.06	aVF -2.60 -1.00	aVF -2.60 -1.00	aVF -1.05 -0.93	V6 0.00 -0.13	V6 -1.95 -1.67	V6 -1.95 -1.67	V6 -0.65 -0.50

FIG. 7.2 A positive exercise stress test (EST) showing horizontal ST depression in L II, L III, aVF and V3–V6 at peak exercise.

perfusion at rest is the hallmark of reversible myocardial ischaemia.

- Symptom-limited exercise is generally the preferred mode of stress in patients who can exercise to a satisfactory workload. This is because exercise can provide higher physiological stress and better correlation between a patient's symptoms and physical work capacity than would be achieved by pharmacological testing.
- Pharmacological stress testing (adenosine, dobutamine) with perfusion scintigraphy is indicated in patients who are unable to exercise adequately or who have left bundle branch block.

Coronary artery calcium scoring

- Coronary artery calcium scoring (CACS) is a non-invasive quantitation of coronary artery calcification using a computed tomography scan. It is a marker of atherosclerotic plaque burden and an independent predictor of future myocardial infarction and mortality.[9]

- CACS is of most value in intermediate-risk patients who are asymptomatic, do not have known CAD and are aged 45–75 years; it is able to reclassify these patients into lower- or higher-risk groups.
- CACS should not be used for high-risk patients, patients with documented CAD or for symptomatic patients.

Computed tomography coronary angiography

- Coronary anatomy may be visualised by computed tomography coronary angiography (CTCA). CTCA provides additional information about the vessel condition, positive or negative remodelling and the presence of plaque surrounding the lumen. These abnormalities are not well demonstrated by invasive coronary angiography, which generally shows only the coronary lumen.
- At a minimum, a 64-slice CT scanner is needed to produce detailed images of the coronary circulation in a non-invasive manner (Fig. 7.3). In symptomatic patients with low to intermediate pretest probability

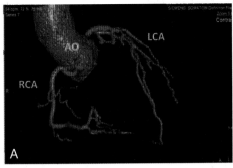 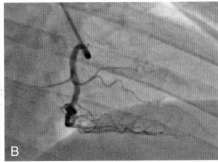

FIG. 7.3 **(A)** A CT coronary angiography (AO=aorta, RCA=right coronary artery, LCA=left coronary artery). **(B)** Coronary angiography of the right coronary artery of the same patient.

of CAD, it has relatively high sensitivity and has been shown to be reliable in ruling out significant CAD.[1,10]

- It should not generally be used in asymptomatic subjects, patients with known significant CAD or patients with a high pretest probability of CAD.
- The radiation dose of CTCA was previously two to three times that of invasive coronary angiography, but with modern protocols it is similar or lower.
- Patients generally need to be in sinus rhythm, tolerate beta-blockers and nitrates, have a heart rate <65 beats per minute, be able to hold their breath for 10 seconds and have a normal renal function. Patients with cardiac arrhythmias, such as atrial fibrillation, may not be successfully imaged with coronary CTCA owing to image degradation from cardiac motion artefact. Similarly, the specificity of CTCA decreases significantly with increasing amount of coronary calcium (Agatston score >400).

Invasive Coronary Angiography

Invasive coronary angiography (ICA) remains the 'gold standard' in depicting epicardial coronary artery disease. However, the imaging information is only about the lumen, and not the plaque. Coronary angiography is an invasive procedure and should be performed only in patients who are amenable to, and candidates for, coronary revascularisstion.[11]

Indication for coronary angiography in stable coronary artery disease

- Coronary angiography is useful in patients with presumed stable CAD who have unacceptable ischaemic symptoms despite guideline-directed medical therapy.
- ICA is also used to define the extent and severity of stable coronary artery disease in patients whose clinical characteristics and for whom the results of

initial non-invasive testing indicate a high likelihood of severe disease.

Complications of coronary angiography

In the hand of an experienced operator, coronary angiography is a safe procedure. Complications are rare and include:

- death – procedural mortality has fallen to 0.1%
- myocardial infarction – the general risk of MI in most series is less than 0.1%
- cerebrovascular accident – the incidence of stroke was found to be 0.07 to 0.10%
- local vascular complications.

The above investigations are summarised in Table 7.3.

PHARMACOLOGICAL MANAGEMENT OF STABLE CORONARY DISEASE

Generally, beta-blockers and calcium channel blockers are the first-line treatment for angina unless contraindicated (see Table 7.2). For second-line treatment it is recommended to add long-acting nitrates, nicorandil or ivabradine. In selective cases perhexiline could be added. Treatment with perhexiline needs monitoring of the drug level. Side effects of perhexiline include neurotoxicity and hepatotoxicity. Fortunately, side effects are rare when drug levels are monitored regularly.

REVASCULARISATION VS MEDICAL THERAPY

Randomised controlled trials comparing revascularisation with optimal medical treatment show that revascularisation generally results in better symptom relief and less need for urgent revascularisation compared with medical treatment, but does not improve mortality.

TABLE 7.3
Investigating Stable Coronary Artery Disease

Test	Indications	Advantages	Disadvantages
Exercise stress test (EST)	Assessment of chest pain in patients with intermediate probability for coronary artery disease	EST is simple, widely available and a low-cost technique; relatively high specificity; functional test	Low sensitivity; no or limited diagnostic value in presence of LBBB, paced rhythm, WPW syndrome, LVH and use of digoxin
Stress echocardiography	Preferred non-invasive imaging technique for assessment of stable coronary artery disease	Low cost, wide availability and lack of radiation exposure; compared with nuclear imaging, stress echocardiography has similar accuracy and markedly higher specificity	Interpretation dependent on operator experiences
Myocardial perfusion scintigraphy using SPECT	Indicated for assessing chest pain in patients who are unable to exercise adequately or who have abnormal baseline ECG (e.g. LBBB)	Provides a more sensitive prediction of the presence of CAD than the exercise stress test	Adenosine may produce bronchospasm in susceptible individuals; thallium-201 is associated with high radiation exposure
Coronary artery calcium scoring (CACS)	Indicated for quantitation of coronary artery calcification, a marker of atherosclerotic plaque burden	Useful in intermediate risk patients who are asymptomatic, to re-classify them into lower or higher risk groups; an independent predictor of future myocardial infarction and mortality	Not useful in high-risk patients, patients with documented CAD and in symptomatic patients
Computed tomography coronary angiography (CTCA)	Useful in low- to intermediate-risk patients when initial exercise test is inconclusive	Provides additional information about the vessel condition, remodelling and plaque surrounding the lumen	Difficult to interpret in presence of coronary calcification, obesity, atrial fibrillation and heart rate >65/min; risk of radiation
Coronary angiography	To define the extent and severity of CAD in patients whose initial non-invasive testing indicates a high likelihood of disease	Remains the 'gold standard' in detecting coronary artery disease	Invasive procedure with the risk of serious complications (stroke, myocardial infarction, death 0.1%); access site complications 5% (less with radial angiography)

CACS=coronary artery calcium scoring; CAD=coronary artery disease; LBBB=left bundle branch block; LVH=left ventricle hypertrophy; SPECT=single photon emission computed tomography; WHW=Wolff–Parkinson–White.

The COURAGE (Clinical Outcomes Utilizing Revascularization and Aggressive Drug Evaluation) trial was a randomised trial involving 2287 patients who had stable coronary artery disease and initial Canadian Cardiovascular Society (CCS) class IV angina (see Table 7.1), subsequently stabilised medically. Entry criteria also included stenosis of at least 70% in at least one proximal epicardial coronary artery and objective evidence of myocardial ischaemia, or at least coronary stenosis of minimally 80% and classic angina without provocative testing. Patients were randomised to undergo angioplasty or to receive optimal medical therapy alone. The primary outcome of death from any cause or non-fatal myocardial infarction did not vary between the two groups during a mean follow-up of 4.6 years.[12]

Similarly, the BARI-2D trial[13] included patients with stable ischaemic heart disease and diabetes, who were randomised to routine revascularisation (in addition to medical treatment) or to a strategy of medical treatment alone. Both percutaneous angioplasty (PCI) and coronary artery bypass graft (CABG) were used for revascularisation. Again, there were no survival benefits of the routine revascularisation strategy for either the PCI patients or the CABG patients. Both studies found an early, significant symptomatic benefit of revascularisation.

The Contemporary trial[14] showed that, in patients with stable coronary artery disease, the presence of significant demonstrable ischaemia as noted by a positive test is important to risk-stratify patients before pursuing PCI. In patients with stable coronary artery disease, fractional flow reserve-guided PCI, as compared with medical therapy alone, improves the outcome.

In the recently released, multicentre ISCHEMIA trial (International Study of Comparative Health Effectiveness with Medical and Invasive Approaches), 5179 patients were randomised to determine the best management strategy for higher-risk patients with stable coronary artery disease who had moderate or severe ischaemia on stress testing.[15] A computed tomography coronary angiogram (CTCA) was performed in most participants to exclude significant left main disease. Eligible patients were then assigned randomly to an initial invasive strategy with coronary angiography followed by revascularisation, when feasible, plus optimal medical therapy or to initial medical therapy alone. An initial invasive approach compared with a conservative approach in stable coronary artery disease patients with moderate–severe ischaemia did not reduce the risk of ischaemic cardiovascular events or death from any cause over a median of 3.2 years.

Dawn continued to get recurrent exertional chest pain despite pharmacological treatment. Her stress echocardiogram was electrically and symptomatically positive at low workload. She also had wall motion abnormalities in the right coronary artery territory at a peak workload. She went on to have a coronary angiogram, which showed an 80% in-stent restenosis of the right coronary artery. She had a stent (drug-eluting) with good results and was discharged home the next day.

REFERENCES

1. Task Force Members, Montalescot G, Sechtem U, Achenbach S, Andreotti F, Arden C, et al. 2013 ESC guidelines on the management of stable coronary artery disease. The Task Force on the management of stable coronary artery disease of the European Society of Cardiology. *Eur Heart J* 2013;**34**:2949–3003.
2. Byrne RA, Joner M, Kastrati A. Stent thrombosis and restenosis: what have we learned and where are we going? The Andreas Gruntzig Lecture ESC 2014. *Eur Heart J* 2015;**36**:3320–31.
3. van Werkum J, Godschalk T, Oirbans T, ten Berg J. Coronary stent thrombosis: incidence, predictors and triggering mechanisms. *Interv Cardiol* 2011;3(5):https://www.openaccessjournals.com/articles/coronary-stent-thrombosis-incidence-predictors-and-triggering-mechanisms.pdf.
4. Wenaweser P, Daemen J, Zwahlen M, van Domburg R, Jüni P, Vaina S, et al. Incidence and correlates of drug-eluting stent thrombosis in routine clinical practice. 4-year results from a large 2-institutional cohort study. *J Am Coll Cardiol* 2008;**52**(14):1134–40.
5. Tada T, Byrne RA, Simunovic I, King LA, Cassese S, Joner M, et al. Risk of stent thrombosis among bare-metal stents, first-generation drug-eluting stents, and second-generation drug-eluting stents: results from a registry of 18,334 patients. *JACC Cardiovasc Interv* 2013;**6**:1267–74.
6. Froelicher VF, Lehmann KG, Thomas R, Goldman S, Morrison D, Edson R, et al. The electrocardiographic exercise test in a population with reduced workup bias: diagnostic performance, computerized interpretation, and multivariable prediction. Veterans Affairs Cooperative Study in Health Services #016 (QUEXTA) Study Group. Quantitative Exercise Testing and Angiography. *Ann Intern Med* 1998;**128**:965–74.
7. Sicariand R, Cortigiani L. The clinical use of stress echocardiography in ischemic heart disease. *Cardiovasc Ultrasound* 2017;**15**:7.
8. Heijenbrok-Kal MH, Fleischmann KE, Hunink MG. Stress echocardiography, stress single-photon-emission computed tomography and electron beam computed tomography for the assessment of coronary artery disease: a meta-analysis of diagnostic performance. *Am Heart J* 2007;**154**:415–23.
9. Hamilton-Craig C, Liew G, Chan J, Chow C, Jelinek M, van Pelt N, et al. *Coronary Artery Calcium Scoring – Position Statement.* Sydney, NSW: The Cardiac Society of Australia and New Zealand. https://www.csanz.edu.au/wp-content/uploads/2017/07/CAC_Position-Statement_2017_ratified-26-May-2017.pdf.
10. Liew GYH, Feneley MP, Worthley SG. Appropriate indications for computed tomography coronary angiography. *Med J Aust* 2012;**196**(4):246–9.
11. Fihn SD, Blankenship JC, Alexander KP, Bittl JA, Byrne JG, Fletcher BJ, et al. 2014 ACC/AHA/AATS/PCNA/SCAI/STS Focused update of the guideline for the diagnosis and management of patients with stable ischemic heart disease. *J Am Coll Cardiol* 2014;**64**(18):1929–49.
12. Boden WE, O'Rourke RA, Teo KK, Hartigan PM, Maron DJ, Kostuk WJ, et al. Optimal medical therapy with or without PCI for stable coronary disease. *N Engl J Med* 2007;**356**:1503–16.

13. Frye RL, August P, Brooks MM, Hardison RM, Kelsey SF, MacGregor JM, et al. A randomized trial of therapies for type 2 diabetes and coronary artery disease. *N Engl J Med* 2009;**360**:2503–15.

14. De Bruyne B, Fearon WF, Pijls NHJ, Barbato E, Tonino P, Piroth Z, et al; the FAME 2 Trial Investigators. Fractional flow reserve–guided PCI for stable coronary artery disease. *N Engl J Med* 2014;**371**:1208–17.

15. Maron DJ, Hochman JS, Reynolds HR, Bangalore S, O'Brien SM, Boden WE, et al; for the ISCHEMIA research group. Initial invasive or conservative strategy for stable coronary disease. *N Engl J Med* 2020;**382**:1395–407.

Sudden Cardiac Death

CASE 10 SCENARIO: PAUL WITH SYSTOLIC MURMUR

Paul, a 28-year-old male, comes to the practice for assessment. He is anxious; his brother died suddenly at the age of 25 while playing soccer 10 days ago. Generally, he is fit and healthy; he works as a builder. He doesn't smoke or drink alcohol. He is not on any medication. Examination reveals a double apical pulse and grade 3/6 ejection systolic murmur loudest in the aortic area that intensifies with the Valsalva manoeuvre.

His ECG shows high QRS voltage, T-wave inversion in most leads (Fig. 8.1).

- Between the calendar years 1985 and 1987, the World Health Organization MONICA project, a population-based register designed to study longitudinal trends within populations, provided the opportunity for relating rates of validated coronary heart disease (CHD) deaths to non-fatal myocardial infarction across populations aged 35 to 64 in 38 different populations. Based on that, in Australia and New Zealand up to 80,000 people die suddenly each year from various causes.[1]
- A more recent study, which prospectively collected information on all cases of sudden cardiac death among children and young adults 1–35 years of age in Australia and New Zealand from 2010 to 2012, found an annual incidence of 1.3 cases per 100,000 persons.[2]

- Sudden cardiac death can have significant emotional and psychological effects on the survivor and immediate family members.
- Although epidemiological risk factors such as age, prior myocardial infarction and low ejection fraction are well established, the syndrome of SCD also has a strong genetic component. Studies demonstrate a marked increase in risk of SCD in first-degree relatives of SCD victims. In the Paris Prospective Study, a parental history of SCD increased the risk of fatal arrhythmia in the offspring by 80%; in subjects with both parents affected, risk of SCD increased ninefold.[3]
- Sudden cardiac death in the young (<35 years) has a structural basis in up to 80% of cases. In young athletes, sudden cardiac death most often occurs in association with hypertrophic cardiomyopathy, and in older athletes in association with CHD.[4]
- HCM, the most common known inherited predisposition to SCD in the young, affects ≈0.5% of the population and may account for as much as 48% of SCD in patients aged <35 years.[5] In addition to these structural heart diseases, a number of electrophysiological diseases and acquired diseases can also cause SCD.

It is important to identify high-risk relatives of SCD victims by taking a careful history and making a detailed cardiovascular examination, an ECG and in selected cases an echocardiograph. In this way, previously unrecognised cardiac conditions can be diagnosed and the incidence of SCD amongst first-degree relatives significantly reduced.

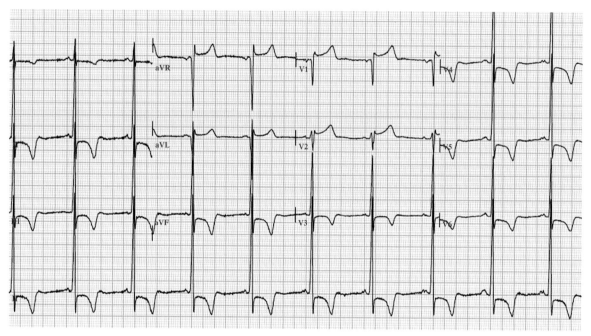

FIG. 8.1 ECG shows high QRS voltage, T-wave inversion in most leads.

On detailed questioning, Paul describes increasing dyspnoea on exertion. He has no history of syncope or presyncope. He denies any history of chest pain or discomfort.

DEFINITION OF SUDDEN CARDIAC DEATH

Sudden cardiac death (SCD) is defined as an unexpected natural death of cardiac cause, heralded by sudden loss of consciousness within 1 hour of symptom onset, in someone without a previously known cardiovascular abnormality.[6] The incidence of SCD in young adults (<35 years old) is estimated at 1.5–5.5 per 100,000 persons per year; however, this includes non-cardiac causes.[7]

AETIOLOGY OF SUDDEN CARDIAC DEATH

In young athletes the cause of SCD may be structural, electrical or acquired.

- The most common structural pathologies are the cardiomyopathies: hypertrophic cardiomyopathy (HCM) (Fig. 8.2), arrhythmogenic right ventricular cardiomyopathy (ARVC) and congenital coronary artery anomalies.
- Primary electrophysiological diseases include Wolff–Parkinson–White syndrome (WPW syndrome), long QT syndrome (LQTS) and Brugada syndrome.
- For athletes who are older than 35, coronary artery disease is the primary cause of death (Fig. 8.3).

Coronary artery disease in athletes younger than 35 can also occur as a result of premature atherosclerosis, usually due to familial hypercholesterolaemia. Other acquired causes may include spontaneous dissection of a coronary artery, myocarditis, etc.

SCD is more common in athletes than in their non-athletic counterparts owing to the increased risk associated with strenuous exercise in the context of a quiescent cardiac abnormality. Data from Italy have shown a 2.8-fold greater risk of SCD among competitive athletes compared with their non-athletic counterparts.[8] There is a significant male predominance of SCD among athletes. Data from the National Center for Catastrophic Sports Injury Research on high school and college athletes reported a 5-fold higher incidence of SCD in male compared with female athletes.[9]

STRUCTURAL CARDIAC ABNORMALITIES
Hypertrophic Cardiomyopathy

- Hypertrophic cardiomyopathy (HCM) is an inherited heart muscle disorder (autosomal dominant) and remains the leading cause of SCD in young athletes in the United States. Its prevalence is estimated at 1:500, with diverse clinical and functional expression ranging from benign to left ventricular outflow tract obstruction (LVOT), myocardial ischaemia and life-threatening arrhythmias with SCD.[10]

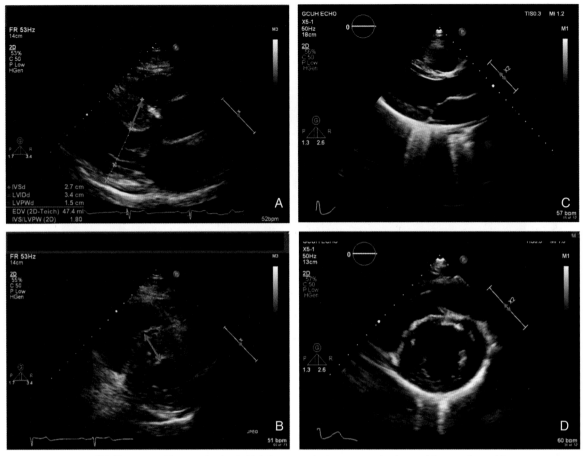

FIG. 8.2 **(A)** (Parasternal long axis view) thick interventricular septum (red arrow) in a patient with hypertrophic cardiomyopathy. **(B)** The same patient in the parasternal short axis view. **(C and D)** The corresponding images in a normal subject.

- SCD has an annual estimated frequency of 2%–4% but is most common in asymptomatic young adults (<30 years old).[11] SCD is likely to be a result of multiple interacting pathologies. Morphologically, myocyte disarray and asymmetric left ventricular hypertrophy (see Fig. 8.2) increase the potential for myocardial ischaemia, and replacement scarring can lead to ventricular arrhythmias and SCD.[12] Risk factors for sudden cardiac death in HCM are shown in Box 8.1.[13]
- SCD can occur in asymptomatic individuals. An important challenge remains in diagnosing such patients and in identifying those at risk of SCD (Table 8.1). Risk factors for SCD include:
  - previous cardiac arrest or sustained ventricular tachycardia (VT)
  - unheralded syncope
  - a family history of SCD

  - intraventricular septum thickness of >30 mm
  - attenuated blood pressure response to exercise.[14]
- Patients may have experienced unexplained syncope and, when detailed questioning reveals recurrent episodes of exertional syncope during childhood or adolescence, this is an ominous sign. However, current evidence suggests that exercise limitation due to chest pain and dyspnoea does not predict SCD.[15]

A typical patient like Paul may have following signs:
1. *a jerky pulse*
2. *a jugular venous pulse (JVP) with a prominent a wave caused by forceful atrial contraction against diminished right ventricular compliance which is secondary to hypertrophy of the ventricular septum*
3. *a double apical impulse which results from a forceful left atrial contraction against a non-compliant left ventricle;*

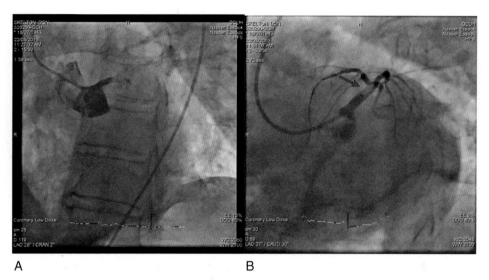

FIG. 8.3 Coronary angiography of a 58-year-old man with resuscitated cardiac arrest showed totally occluded left main coronary artery, which was successfully stented **(A)**. His initial ECG showed anterior ST elevation **(B)**. Arrow indicates a large thrombus in the distal left main artery.

BOX 8.1
Risk for Sudden Cardiac Death in Hypertrophic Cardiomyopathy[13]

- Prior cardiac arrest
- History of recurrent syncope and family history of sudden cardiac death
- Presence of non-sustained ventricular tachycardia during ambulatory ECG monitoring
- Abnormal exercise blood pressure response; a rise in systolic blood pressure from baseline to peak exercise of <25 mmHg
- Severe left ventricular hypertrophy; the left ventricular wall thickness in any myocardial segment of ≥30 mm in two-dimensional echocardiography
- Left ventricular outflow tract obstruction with resting peak instantaneous outflow tract gradient >30 mmHg

---

a fourth heart sound is frequently heard because atrial systole occurs against a non-compliant left ventricle

4. *a loud ejection systolic murmur which increases with Valsalva manoeuvre (a result of increased outflow tract obstruction due to decreased left ventricular end diastolic volume with increased intrathoracic pressure)*

5. *a pansystolic murmur at the apex and axilla due to mitral regurgitation – a result of systolic anterior motion (SAM) of the mitral valve, which is a feature of hypertrophic cardiomyopathy.*

- The diagnosis is made using ECG and echocardiography. More than 90% of affected individuals have an abnormal resting ECG. ECG abnormalities may include: voltage criteria for left ventricular enlargement, left atrial enlargement, left axis deviation, ST segment depression, T-wave inversion and pathological Q waves.[12]
- Echocardiography may reveal septal hypertrophy, which is associated with an increased risk of SCD.[16] Cardiac hypertrophy is generally asymmetrical. There may also be systolic anterior motion of the mitral valve and a left ventricular outflow tract gradient. Important differential diagnoses include hypertensive heart disease and athlete's heart. Unlike HCM, hypertensive heart disease generally causes concentric hypertrophy and the maximum wall thickness is generally mild.
- Contrast-enhanced cardiac MRI may help to provide more-accurate left ventricular wall thickness measurements and risk stratification.
- Cardiac arrest, from ventricular tachycardia or fibrillation, may be the first clinical manifestation of the disease. Patients who survive have a subsequent annual mortality from SCD of 4%.[17]

TABLE 8.1
Common Causes of Sudden Cardiac Death

Structural cardiac abnormalities	Hypertrophic cardiomyopathy (HCM)	Autosomal dominant; sudden death can be the first clinical manifestation; examination may reveal a loud systolic murmur which increases with Valsalva manoeuvre; more than 90% of affected individuals have an abnormal ECG.
	Arrhythmogenic right ventricular cardiomyopathy (ARVC)	Progressive fibro-fatty replacement of the (R) ventricle with dilation; T-wave inversion in V1–V3, RBBB pattern, ε wave (a small positive deflection buried in the end of the QRS complex), ventricular ectopy of LBBB morphology.
	Congenital coronary artery anomaly (CCAA)	The most common anomalies include origin of the left coronary artery from the right sinus of Valsalva and right coronary artery origin from the left sinus of Valsalva; SCD results from ventricular arrhythmia triggered by myocardial ischaemia during exercise.
Primary electrophysiological disease	Wolff–Parkinson–White syndrome (WPW)	The incidence of WPW is between 0.1% and 0.3% in the general population; SCD is usually caused by the propagation of atrial fibrillation to the ventricles by the accessory pathway with a very rapid ventricular response rate; the ECG may reveal a δ wave and short P–R interval.
	Long QT syndrome (LQTS)	Can lead to syncope and sudden death by means of polymorphic ventricular tachycardia; the ECG typically reveals a heart-rate-corrected Q–T interval >460 ms in women and >440 ms in men.
	Brugada syndrome	This is an autosomal dominant condition; SCD often occurs during sleep; There is an RBBB pattern with coved ST elevation over the right precordial leads of V1–V3.
Acquired cardiac abnormalities	Atherosclerotic coronary artery disease (CAD)	CAD is the primary cause of sudden death in patients >35 years of age; younger patients (<35 years) with familial hypercholesterolaemia can also die suddenly from CAD.
	Myocarditis	There may be a history of viral illness; there is often abnormal conduction in the ECG and troponin elevation; wall motion abnormalities may be seen in the echocardiogram.
	Illicit drugs/performance-enhancing drugs	Can be associated with cardiomyopathy, hypertension and SCD; a toxicology screen may be helpful.

LBBB=left bundle branch block; RBBB=right bundle branch block.

Arrhythmogenic Right Ventricular Cardiomyopathy

- Arrhythmogenic right ventricular cardiomyopathy (ARVC) is characterised by regional and global fibro-fatty replacement of the right and, less commonly, left ventricular myocardium, with electrical instability and the risk of SCD as a result of ventricular arrhythmias.
- It is an inherited condition, with an estimated 1 : 1000–1 : 10,000 prevalence, and has been thought to account for approximately 25% of SCD in young athletes.[18]

- Generally, examination findings are unremarkable, but careful interpretation of electrocardiogram may show inverted T waves and prolonged QRS complex with ε waves (a small positive deflection buried in the end of the QRS complex) in the right precordial leads.
- Strenuous exercise and acute mental stress are the major triggering mechanisms for SCD. It is postulated

increased afterload stretches the diseased myocardium and catecholamine interaction with a 'supersensitive' myocardium contributes to the ventricular arrhythmias.[19]

- Patients with sustained monomorphic ventricular tachycardia are thought to have a more favourable prognosis when treated medically with sotalol.[20] In patients with aborted SCD or VT refractory to medical therapy an implanted cardioverter defibrillator (ICD) is indicated.

Congenital Coronary Artery Anomaly

- Congenital coronary artery anomalies (CCAAs) are rare. The estimated prevalence is 0.3%–1.2% in patients referred for coronary angiography.
- The anomalies most responsible for SCD include the origin of the left coronary artery from the non-coronary aortic left sinus of Valsalva or from the right sinus, especially when the artery travels between the aortic and pulmonary roots.[21] Myocardial ischaemia is precipitated by impaired coronary blood flow from compression between the great vessels, coronary spasm from endothelial dysfunction, or the abnormal slit-like ostium of the anomalous coronary artery compromising flow reserve.[22]
- SCD may be the first manifestation of CCAA and clinicians must have a high index of suspicion in young patients who present with either exertional chest pain or syncope with unexplained QRS or ST–T-wave changes detected after successful resuscitation. Surgical intervention should be recommended for these patients when they are thought to have a high risk of SCD.

OTHER STRUCTURAL HEART ABNORMALITIES

Other structural cardiac abnormalities associated with SCD in young individuals include aortic dissection, typically in the context of Marfan syndrome, mitral valve prolapse and bicuspid aortic valve with aortic stenosis.

Primary Electrophysiological Disease
Wolff–Parkinson–White syndrome

- Wolff–Parkinson–White (WPW) syndrome induces paroxysmal arrhythmias due to an accessory pathway with anterograde conduction causing ventricle pre-excitation.
- Patients are usually asymptomatic but may complain of palpitations occurring with tachyarrhythmia.
- SCD is characteristically a result of the development of atrial fibrillation (AF), which is itself more common

in WPW patients. The short anterograde refractory period of the accessory pathway means very rapid ventricular response rates may occur and degenerate into ventricular fibrillation (VF) and SCD. Population-based studies suggest an incidence of SCD of 0.15% per year.[23]

- The ECG characteristically shows a short P–R interval (<120 ms), a δ wave (slurring of the initial portion of the QRS complex), QRS prolongation, ST–T-wave changes and a pseudoinfarction pattern (Q waves).[a]
- Risk factors associated with development of sudden cardiac death include: male gender, a demonstrated very rapid ventricular rate during AF due to short refractory periods of the accessory pathway, a history of previous AF, and the presence of multiple accessory pathways.[24]
- Electrophysiology studies are important for determining the electrical properties of the accessory pathway for risk stratification and referral for catheter ablation.

Long QT syndrome

- Long QT syndrome (LQTS) is a disorder of cardiac repolarisation; it is characterised by a prolonged Q–T interval on ECG and an increased risk of sudden death. LQTS can be subdivided into congenital or acquired.
- The acquired form can develop in response to a variety of conditions associated with QT prolongation, including drugs and electrolyte disturbances.
- Long QT is defined as a corrected Q–T interval of ≥440 ms and ≥460 ms in men and women respectively.[25]
- Long QT can lead to syncope and sudden death as a result of polymorphic ventricular tachycardia, which can deteriorate to VF. A younger age of occurrence of the first syncope predicts a poor outcome. The degree of QT prolongation is also associated with increased risk. A QT of more than 500 ms predisposes to *torsades de pointes* and VF.[26] Symptoms are frequently precipitated by adrenergic stress such as physical exertion or emotion.
- Romano–Ward syndrome, a familial autosomal dominant condition, and Jarvell and Lang–Neilsen syndrome, a familial autosomal recessive condition with congenital deafness, are both recognised as LQTSs with a more severe prognosis.
- All patients with LQTS, whether asymptomatic or symptomatic, should reduce physical stress and avoid

---

[a]The presence of the ECG changes is called 'WPW conduction'. Patients with WPW conduction and episodes of supraventricular tachycardia have 'Wolff–Parkinson–White syndrome'.

any drugs that prolong repolarisation. Only retrospective data are available to support the role of beta-blockers. The obvious clinical efficacy of beta-blockers makes a randomised trial difficult to justify. A retrospective study of 233 patients by Schwartz showed a 15% mortality following the first syncope in patients treated with beta-blockers, left cardiac sympathetic denervation or both, compared with a 60% mortality in patients not treated or on miscellaneous therapy.[27] An implantable cardioverter defibrillator is indicated for patients who have been resuscitated from a cardiac arrest.

Brugada syndrome

- Brugada syndrome is an arrhythmogenic disorder of a structurally normal heart. Patients present with syncope due to polymorphic ventricular tachycardia or SCD from VF.[28]
- Electrocardiography characteristically reveals a partial right bundle branch block and ST elevation in leads V1–V3.
- At 3 years follow-up, cardiac arrest in both symptomatic and asymptomatic patients has been shown to be 30% with SCD usually occurring at rest or during sleep and in the third or fourth decade of life.[29] It is recommended that survivors of cardiac arrest have an ICD.

Acquired Cardiac Abnormalities

- Myocarditis, most often caused by viral infections, accounts for up to 7% of SCD in athletes.[30] The diagnosis of myocarditis should be considered in any healthy young individual with a recent viral illness and cardiac symptoms. There may be new abnormal ECG changes and regional wall motion abnormalities on echocardiography.
- Blunt trauma to the chest wall can trigger ventricular fibrillation and SCD without causing direct injury to the thoracic cage or heart.[31]
- The use of performance-enhancing drugs, including anabolic–androgenic steroids, is known to cause SCD in young individuals and its use may be underestimated.
- As mentioned above, SCD in the young can also result from premature atherosclerotic coronary artery disease. It is most commonly a manifestation of familial hypercholesterolaemia.

Paul was referred to cardiology for an echocardiogram and was subsequently diagnosed with HCM. He had a 24-hour Holter monitor, which revealed episodes of self-limiting ventricular tachycardia lasting up to 20 seconds. His exercise test was also associated with brief episodes of VT at high levels of exercise. After discussion and explanation an ICD was recommended and he was advised not to play competitive sport. Eighteen months after his ICD was inserted, he received an appropriate shock from the device for an episode of rapid VT which occurred during exercise. His other family members were recommended to have screening tests.

REFERENCES

1. Tunstall-Pedoe H, Kuulasmaa K, Amouyel P, Arveiler D, Rajakangas AM, Pajak A. Myocardial infarction and coronary deaths in the World Health Organization MONICA Project: registration procedures, event rates, and case-fatality rates in 38 populations from 21 countries in four continents. *Circulation* 1994;**90**:583–612.
2. Bagnall RD, Weintraub RG, Ingles J, Duflou J, Yeates L, Lam L, et al. A prospective study of sudden cardiac death among children and young adults. *N Engl J Med* 2016;**374**:2441–52.
3. Jouven X, Desnos M, Guerot C, Ducimetiere P. Predicting sudden death in the population: the Paris Prospective Study I. *Circulation* 1999;**99**:1978–83.
4. Maron BJ, Shirani J, Poliac LC, Mathenge R, Roberts WC, Mueller FO. Sudden death in young competitive athletes: clinical, demographic, and pathological profiles. *JAMA* 1996;**276**:199–204.
5. Zipes DP, Wellens HJ. Sudden cardiac death. *Circulation* 1998;**98**:2334–51.
6. Myerburg RJ, Castellanos A. Cardiac arrest and sudden cardiac death. In: Braunwald E, editor. *Heart disease: a textbook of cardiovascular medicine.* New York: WB Saunders; 1997. pp. 742–79.
7. Sen-Chowdhry S, McKenna WJ. Sudden cardiac death in the young: strategy for prevention by targeted evaluation. *Cardiology* 2006;**105**:196–206.
8. Corrado D, Basso C, Rizzoli G, Schiavon M, Thiene G. Does sports activity enhance the risk of sudden death in adolescents and young adults? *J Am Coll Cardiol* 2003;**42**:1959–63.
9. Van Camp SP, Bloor C, Mueller FO, Cantu R, Olson H. Nontraumatic sports death in high school and college athletes. *Med Sci Sports Exerc* 1995;**27**:641–7.
10. Maron BJ. Hypertrophic cardiomyopathy. *Lancet* 1997;**350**: 127–33.
11. McKenna W, Deanfield J, Faruqui A, England D, Oakley C, Goodwin J. Prognosis in hypertrophic cardiomyopathy: role of age and clinical, electrocardiographic and haemodynamic features. *Am J Cardiol* 1981;**47**:532–8.
12. Spirito P, Seidman CE, McKenna WJ, Maron BJ. The management of hypertrophic cardiomyopathy. *N Engl J Med* 1997;**336**:775–85.
13. Frenneaux MP. Assessing the risk of sudden cardiac death in a patient with hypertrophic cardiomyopathy. *Heart* 2004;**90**:570–5.
14. Chandra N, Bastiaenen R, Papadakis M, Sharma S. Sudden cardiac death in young athletes: practical challenges and diagnostic dilemmas. *J Am Coll Cardiol* 2013;**61**(10):1027–40.

15. Sharma S, Elliott P, Whyte G, Mahon N, Virdee MS, Mist B, et al. Utility of cardio-pulmonary exercise in the assessment of clinical determinants of functional capacity in hypertrophic cardiomyopathy. *J Am Coll Cardiol* 2000;**86**:162–8.

16. Spirito P, Bellone P, Harris KM, Bernabo P, Bruzzi P, Maron BJ. Magnitude of left ventricular hypertrophy and risk of sudden death in hypertrophic cardiomyopathy. *N Engl J Med* 2000;**342**:1778–85.

17. Elliott PM, Sharma S, Varnava A, Poloniecki J, Rowland E, McKenna WJ. Survival after cardiac arrest or sustained ventricular tachycardia in patients with hypertrophic cardiomyopathy. *J Am Coll Cardiol* 1999;**33**:1596–601.

18. Goodin JC, Farb A, Smialek JE, Field F, Virmani R. Right ventricular dysplasia associated with sudden death in young adults. *Mod Pathol* 1991;**4**:702–6.

19. Marcus F, Nava A, Thienne G. *Arrhythmogenic right ventricular cardiomyopathy/dysplasia: recent advances.* Milan: Springer; 2007.

20. Wichter T, Borggrefe M, Haverkamp W, Chen X, Breithardt G. Efficacy of antiarrhythmic drugs in patients with arrhythmogenic right ventricular disease. Results in patients with inducible and noninducible ventricular tachycardia. *Circulation* 1992;**86**:29–37.

21. Kimbiris D, Iskandrian AS, Segal BL, Bemis CE. Anomalous aortic origin of coronary arteries. *Circulation* 1978;**58**:606–15.

22. Angelina P. Coronary artery anomalies. An entity in search of an identity. *Circulation* 2007;**115**:1296–305.

23. Goudevenos JA, Katsouras CS, Graekas G, Argiri O, Giogiakas V, Sideris DA. Ventricular pre-excitation in the general population: a study on the mode of presentation and clinical course. *Heart* 2000;**83**:29–34.

24. Wellens HJ. When to perform catheter ablation in asymptomatic patients with a Wolff–Parkinson–White electrocardiogram. *Circulation* 2005;**112**:2201–16.

25. Moss AG. Prolonged QT-interval syndrome. *JAMA* 1986;**256**:2985–7.

26. Moss AJ, Schwartz PJ, Crampton RS, Tzivoni D, Locati EH, MacCluer J, et al. The long QT syndrome. Prospective longitudinal study of 328 families. *Circulation* 1991;**84**:1136–44.

27. Schwartz PJ. Idiopathic long QT syndrome: progress and questions. *Am Heart J* 1985;**109**:399–411.

28. Brugada P, Brugada J. Right bundle branch block, persistent ST segment elevation and sudden cardiac death: a distinct clinical and electrocardiographic syndrome. A multicenter report. *J Am Coll Cardiol* 1992;**20**:1391–6.

29. Priori SG, Aliot E, Blomstrom-Lundqvist C, Bossaert L, Breithardt G, Brugada P, et al. Update of the guidelines on sudden cardiac death of the European Society of Cardiology. *Eur Heart J* 2003;**24**:13–15.

30. Eckart RE, Scoville SL, Campbell CL, Shry EA, Stajduhar KC, Potter RN, et al. Sudden death in young adults: a 25-year review of autopsies in military recruits. *Ann Intern Med* 2004;**141**:829–34.

31. Maron BJ, Gohman TE, Kyle SB, Estes NAM, Link MS. Clinical profile and spectrum of commotio cordis. *JAMA* 2002;**287**:1142–6.

CHAPTER 9

Pericarditis

> **KEY POINTS**
>
> - Pericarditis is a common disease, diagnosed in 5% of patients presenting to the emergency department with chest pain.
> - Clinical diagnosis is made by the presence of characteristic chest pain symptoms, ECG findings and the presence of a pericardial friction rub.
> - It is most commonly of viral or idiopathic origin.
> - Pericarditis of viral and idiopathic aetiology generally has a brief and benign course.
> - Non-steroidal anti-inflammatory drugs (NSAIDs) and colchicine remain the mainstay of treatment for pericarditis.
> - Cardiac tamponade is a serious complication of pericarditis; it can be diagnosed clinically by the presence of decreased blood pressure, elevated jugular venous pressure, muffled heart sounds on auscultation, and pulsus paradoxus.

CASE 11 SCENARIO: DAVID WITH CHEST PAIN

David is a previously fit and healthy 32-year-old male who has presented to the hospital with chest pain that is worse on inspiration.

Chest pain is a common presenting symptom and pericarditis is an important differential diagnosis of chest pain. It is diagnosed in 5% in patients presenting to the emergency department with non-acute myocardial infarction related chest pain.[1]

CLINICAL ASSESSMENT OF CHEST PAIN

The initial clinical assessment should include:
- The history, with an emphasis on the patient's description of the chest pain and the presence of associated symptoms. Risk factors for the important differential diagnosis – ischaemic heart disease – should be assessed. These include: a history of cardiovascular disease, renal impairment, diabetes, hypertension, dyslipidaemia, a positive family history of cardiac disease in first-degree relatives, and smoking.
- Physical examination focusing on the cardiorespiratory system. Important findings may include signs of shock (clamminess, tachycardia, decreased blood pressure), pulsus paradoxus, elevated jugular venous pressure (JVP), changes in heart or lung sounds, and peripheral oedema. Respiratory and localised musculoskeletal

and abdominal examinations are also likely to be indicated.
- Basic investigations including an electrocardiogram (ECG) and chest x-ray (CXR). The need for further testing, including blood tests such as troponin assay or C-reactive protein (CRP), can often be guided by the clinical findings and ECG.

Common Conditions That Cause Chest Pain

The differential diagnosis of chest pain is shown in Box 9.1.

David stated that his pain was retrosternal, sharp and worse on inspiration. It had a sudden onset, did not radiate anywhere and was not associated with any shortness of breath. It was relieved slightly when he sat up and leaned forwards. David did not have any cardiac risk factors and had no past medical conditions except for a recent 'flu-like' illness. He had no risk factors for acquisition of human immunodeficiency virus (HIV) or tuberculosis, or any history of chronic kidney disease.

On clinical examination, David was afebrile and, except for a soft pericardial friction rub, there were no other positive findings.

Clinical Features of Pericarditis
- Pericarditis often presents with sharp retrosternal pain (present in 98.3% of cases) that may or may not radiate to the neck, shoulder or arms.[3] The pain is

> BOX 9.1
> List of Common Conditions That Cause
> Chest Pain[2]
>
> **LIFE-THREATENING CAUSES OF CHEST PAIN**
> - Myocardial infarction
> - Aortic dissection
> - Acute pulmonary embolism
> - Pericarditis with pericardial effusion
> - Pneumothorax
>
> **OTHER COMMON CAUSES**
> - Musculoskeletal/chest wall disease or injury
> - Gastro-oesophageal reflux disease
> - Pulmonary cause
> - Psychogenic/psychosomatic causes
> - Takotsubo cardiomyopathy (stress cardiomyopathy)

often worse when the patient is supine and improves when the patient sits upright or leans forwards. It may be aggravated by deep breathing, swallowing or coughing.

- The pericardial friction rub is the most important physical sign of acute pericarditis (present in 35% of cases).[3] It is a high-pitched, scratching sound and is heard most frequently at the left lower sternal border during expiration with the patient upright and leaning forward. Other important clinical signs to look for are fever >38°C and signs of tamponade (elevated JVP,[a] muffled heart sounds and decreased blood pressure).
- Acute pericarditis is generally diagnosed with at least two of the following criteria: typical chest pain described above, a pericardial friction rub, suggestive changes on the ECG and new or worsening pericardial effusion.
- Other life-threatening causes of chest pain symptoms similar to that of acute pericarditis include pulmonary embolus (often associated with the sudden onset of shortness of breath) and acute myocardial infarction (AMI). An immediate ECG should be performed to look for the characteristic features of these conditions. If the diagnosis is unclear, the patient should be sent to hospital for further assessment and testing (e.g.

coronary angiogram for myocardial infarction and CT pulmonary angiography for suspected pulmonary embolism). Troponin levels may be elevated in all the above conditions, and if a serious condition is suspected the patient should be transferred to the hospital without waiting for the troponin result.

- Pericarditis preceded by viral respiratory or gastro-intestinal symptoms is suggestive of a viral aetiology. Most cases of pericarditis of viral and idiopathic aetiologies are self-limiting and respond rapidly to anti-inflammatory treatment. Risk factors that suggest non-idiopathic, non-viral causes of pericarditis include: fever >38°C (bacterial pericarditis), kidney disease (uraemic pericarditis), unsafe sexual practices and intravenous drug use (HIV pericarditis), history of malignancy (malignant pericarditis), autoimmune disease (lupus or rheumatoid pericarditis) and history of tuberculosis or residence in an area with high prevalence of tuberculosis (tuberculosis pericarditis). Suspicion of a non-viral non-idiopathic aetiology of the pericarditis should prompt referral for a review by a cardiologist.

David's ECG is shown in Fig. 9.1. His chest x-ray was unremarkable. He had mild leukocytosis. His other blood cell counts, electrolytes and troponin were normal. His CRP was mildly elevated.

INVESTIGATING CHEST PAIN
Stages of Development of ECG Changes in Pericarditis

Findings in pericarditis can include PR depression and diffuse ST elevation with upward concavity (acute myocardial infarction typically produces ST elevation with upward convexity) (see Fig. 9.1). The ST elevation usually involves more than one coronary vascular territory and there is an absence of reciprocal ST changes between leads III and aVL. The stages of development of the ECG changes are shown in Table 9.1.[4]

Chest X-ray

- Chest radiography is performed primarily to rule out pericardial effusion and abnormalities in the mediastinum or lung fields that may be responsible for the pericardial effusion (e.g. lung carcinoma). A CXR is also helpful in excluding other causes of chest pain (e.g. pneumothorax).
- The CXR may be normal in presence of a small pericardial effusion (<250 mL).
- A large cardiac silhouette with predominantly an increase in transverse diameter (globular or

---

[a]This may include a positive Kussmaul sign. The JVP rises with inspiration. It strongly suggests the presence of cardiac tamponade.

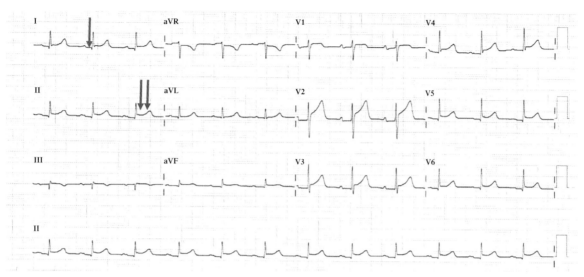

FIG. 9.1 Diffuse upwardly concave ST-segment elevation (double arrow) and PR depression (single arrow) in pericarditis.

TABLE 9.1
Stages of Development of ECG Changes in Pericarditis

Stage	ECG Change	
I	Diffuse ST-segment elevation (double arrows) and PR-segment depression (single arrow)	
II	Normalisation of the ST segment and PR segment	
III	Widespread T-wave inversions (single arrow)	
IV	Normalisation of the T waves	

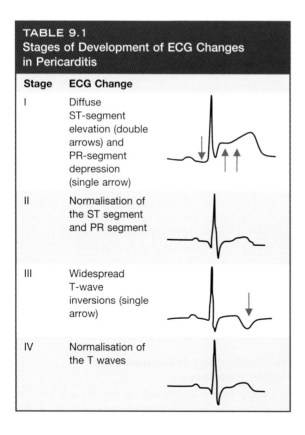

water-bottle shape) is typical of a pericardial effusion (Fig. 9.2). Unlike the increased cardiac silhouette in heart failure, in pericardial effusion the lung fields generally appear clear. Comparisons with the old film are very helpful in detecting an increased cardiac silhouette.

Other Investigations

- Blood tests may reveal leukocytosis. CRP is usually elevated in patients with acute pericarditis; however, it does not have a high specificity for the diagnosis.
- A troponin rise is detectable in more than 30% of cases, as inflammation of the epicardium can lead to troponin release. However, unlike the situation in acute coronary syndromes, elevated troponin in pericarditis is not a negative prognostic marker.[5]

On the basis of his clinical findings, recent viral infection and low risk for ischaemic heart disease, David was diagnosed with viral pericarditis. His symptoms improved with 400 mg oral ibuprofen four times daily.

MANAGEMENT OF PERICARDITIS

- NSAIDs are the mainstay of treatment. Depending on the severity of the symptoms and rapidity of response, ibuprofen 300–800 mg every 6–8 hours

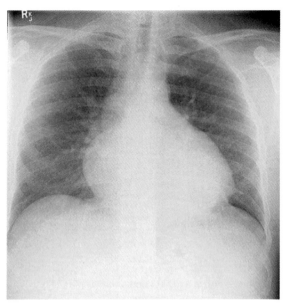

FIG. 9.2 Chest x-ray showing a globular heart shadow, typically seen in pericardial effusion.

may be initially required; it can be continued for 1–2 weeks for an uncomplicated episode and for up to several months for recurrences. CRP should be considered as a marker of disease activity to guide management and treatment length. Gastrointestinal protection with a proton-pump inhibitor (PPI) may need to be considered.[6]

• It is now common practice to use colchicine, in addition to conventional anti-inflammatory therapy for the first episode of pericarditis, unless there are specific contraindications. Generally, colchicine is continued 0.5 mg twice daily, or 0.5 mg daily for patients <70 kg, for 3 months for acute pericarditis.[6,7]

• The ICAP trial (Investigation on Colchicine for Acute Pericarditis), a randomised trial of colchicine versus placebo for acute pericarditis, showed that the addition of colchicine to conventional anti-inflammatory therapy reduced the rate of recurrent pericarditis by more than 50%.[7]

• The CORP trial (Colchicine Prevents Recurrent Pericarditis) was the first multicentre, double-blind randomised trial of colchicine in the secondary prevention of pericarditis. It confirmed that colchicine, when given in addition to conventional therapy, prevents recurrent episodes of pericarditis.[8]

• Colchicine concentrates in leucocytes, disrupts microtubules and prevents chemotaxis that may help

to disrupt the inflammatory cycle involved in the pathogenesis of pericarditis.

• Colchicine is usually well tolerated. Diarrhoea is the major side effect associated with colchicine. It is usually dose dependent and generally reported in fewer than 10% of patients.

• The role of systemic corticosteroids in pericarditis is controversial. High-dose corticosteroids (i.e. prednisone 1 mg/kg per day) with a 2–4-week taper can be considered in pericarditis secondary to connective tissue disease, uraemia or autoreactivity.

Two weeks later, David presented to the hospital complaining of chest discomfort and dizziness on exertion. Clinical examination revealed muffled heart sounds and decreased blood pressure. The JVP was elevated and there was pulsus paradoxus of 25 mmHg. The Kussmaul sign was positive.

Clinical Signs of Pericardial Effusion

Clinical manifestations of pericardial effusion are dependent upon the rate of accumulation of fluid in the pericardial sac. Rapid accumulation of a small amount of pericardial fluid may cause symptomatic elevation of intrapericardial pressures, while large but slowly progressing effusions can be asymptomatic.

• The classic triad of pericardial tamponade includes dilated neck veins, a fall in blood pressure, and muffled heart sounds. There is almost always tachycardia. Other clinical findings of pericardial effusion are shown in Table 9.2.

Assessment of Cardiac Tamponade

• The ECG may show electrical alternans in cardiac tamponade (Fig. 9.3). It is an alternation in the amplitude of QRS complexes and is thought to be due to the swinging movement of the heart within the pericardial cavity. The combination of low-voltage QRS complexes (≤5 mm) in limb leads and tachycardia should always raise concern about tamponade. Other causes of this combination include chronic obstructive pulmonary disease and pleural effusion.

• Urgent referral for echocardiography is important for confirming the presence and size of an effusion. Tamponade is a life-threatening illness. In circumstances where the clinical signs are not definite, echocardiography should be used to look for possible cardiac tamponade.

Mechanism and Measurement of Pulsus Paradoxus

• During inspiration, the negative intrathoracic pressure increases resulting in increased venous return to the

TABLE 9.2
Clinical Signs in the Diagnosis of Pericardial Effusion

System	Clinical Sign
Cardiovascular	1. Pulsus paradoxus is an exaggeration of physiological respiratory variation in systemic blood pressure, defined as a decrease in systolic blood pressure of more than 10 mmHg with inspiration, due to reduced cardiac output during inspiration 2. Kussmaul sign is a rise in JVP on inspiration; it is seen in conditions in which right ventricular filling is limited by pericardial fluid, and in non-compliant pericardium or myocardium 3. Tachycardia 4. Hepatojugular reflux: this can be observed by applying pressure to the periumbilical region. A rise in the JVP of greater than 3 cm H_2O for more than 30 seconds suggests elevated central venous pressure (transient elevation in JVP can be normal) 5. Pericardial rub
Respiratory	1. Tachypnoea 2. Decreased breath sounds
Abdominal	Hepatosplenomegaly
Other	1. Weakened peripheral pulses 2. Oedema 3. Cyanosis

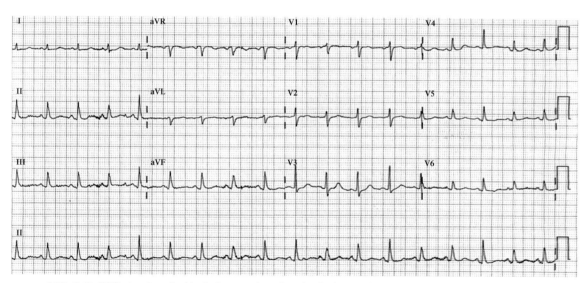

FIG. 9.3 ECG showing electrical alternans (an alteration in the amplitude of the QRS complex), best demonstrated in LII.

heart. The right ventricle distends causing the interventricular septum to bulge into the left ventricle. This results in a decrease in the left ventricular end diastolic volume, thus decreasing stroke volume and arterial pressure during systole. As intrapericardial

pressures rise, this effect becomes pronounced. The converse is true for expiration.

• The sphygmomanometer cuff is inflated above systolic pressure. Korotkoff sounds are sought over the brachial artery while the cuff is deflated slowly.

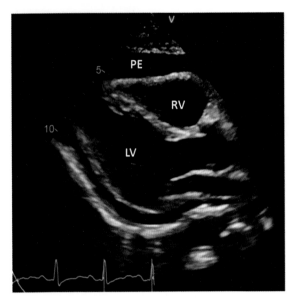

FIG. 9.4 Transthoracic echocardiogram showing pericardial effusion (RV=right ventricle, LV=left ventricle, PE=pericardial effusion).

Initial Korotkoff sounds are heard only during expiration. The cuff is then deflated slowly to establish the pressure at which Korotkoff sounds become audible during both inspiration and expiration. When the differences between these two levels exceeds 10 mmHg during quiet respiration, a paradoxical pulse is present.

An ECG and CXR were performed for David. Initial blood tests were similar to those of his first presentation. David was admitted and a transthoracic echocardiogram was performed, which showed up to 23 mm pericardial effusion with early tamponade (Fig. 9.4).

- A large heart silhouette on CXR is most often due to pericardial effusion. Other common causes of a large heart silhouette include dilated cardiomyopathy.

Complications of Acute Pericarditis

- Complications of acute pericarditis include pericardial effusion (present in 60% of cases), tamponade (5% of cases), myopericarditis and recurrent pericarditis.[1]
- Pericardial effusion is the abnormal accumulation of fluid in the pericardial cavity. Cardiac tamponade occurs when this fluid accumulates under pressure and obstructs diastolic filling of the heart.

- Myopericarditis is another possibly serious complication, with extension of the inflammation to the myocardium, which can be associated with creatinine kinase and troponin elevations and regional wall motion abnormalities on the ECG.
- Constrictive pericarditis is characterised by loss of normal elasticity of the pericardial sac owing to fibrosis, typically as a result of chronic pericardial inflammation.

Pericardiocentesis was performed on David and 900 mL of blood-stained fluid were successfully drained. David's symptoms were relieved, and he recovered over the following day. He was discharged on oral colchicine and ibuprofen and for a follow-up echocardiogram 10 days later.

Pericardiocentesis

- Definitive management for cardiac tamponade includes prompt referral to a hospital where the patient can receive ultrasound or CT guided pericardiocentesis. Pericardiocentesis is indicated for effusions that are moderate to large and are symptomatic, where medical management has been unsuccessful or where pericardial fluid is needed for diagnostic purposes. Prompt pericardiocentesis in cases of pericardial tamponade may be lifesaving.

David's 10-day follow-up transthoracic echocardiogram showed an asymptomatic re-accumulation of 1.7 cm of fluid. At this appointment, further tests were ordered including tumour markers (alpha-fetoprotein, carcinoembryonic antigen (CEA) and carcinoma antigen (CA) 15.3), pericardial fluid cultures for tuberculosis and pericardial fluid cytology. These were negative. Computerised tomography (CT) scan of the abdomen and chest did not show malignancy or lymphadenopathy, and HIV serology was negative. David was also investigated for autoimmune disease. However, other than a mild non-specific elevation in antinuclear antibodies (ANA), autoimmune markers (ENA, pANCA, cANCA, dsDNA) were negative.

Causes of Pericardial Effusion

Recurrence of haemorrhagic effusion is worrying, and when it occurs it is important to exclude serious causes of pericardial effusion such as malignancy, tuberculosis and HIV. As malignancy is a common cause of recurrent haemorrhagic pericarditis, a pericardial tissue biopsy was considered. A negative pericardial fluid cytology for malignant cells does not completely exclude a malignancy. Other causes of pericardial effusion are described in Table 9.3.

TABLE 9.3
Causes of Pericarditis/Pericardial Effusion

Cause		Test
Idiopathic	Most common	Often relates to the lack of extensive diagnostic evaluation; many patients with idiopathic pericarditis have a viral infection
Infectious:		
Viral/HIV	Most common cause of infectious pericarditis. Common organisms include coxsackie virus A and B and echovirus. The pericarditis may be preceded by a prodrome of upper respiratory symptoms.	A fourfold rise in viral antibody titre; serological test for HIV in high-risk patients
Bacterial	May occur following pneumonia, fever ≥38°C	
Tuberculosis	The aetiological spectrum of pericarditis is different in developing countries, with a high prevalence of tuberculosis (up to 70%–80% of pericarditis in sub-Saharan Africa)	Chest radiography, tuberculin test, histology, cultures
Autoimmune disease	Rheumatoid arthritis, lupus	Rheumatoid factor, complement levels, antinuclear antibodies
Neoplastic	Malignancies with the highest prevalence of pericardial effusion include lung (37%), breast (22%) and leukaemia/lymphoma (17%)	Chest radiography, pericardial fluid cytology, tumour markers, haemorrhagic effusion
Postoperative	Common after cardiac surgery	History, evidence of polyserositis, high ESR
Following MI	Often associated with a large anterior myocardial infarction	History, echocardiography
Aortic dissection	Rare	Trans-oesophageal echocardiography, CT aortogram, MRI
Uraemia	Patients with chronic kidney disease before or after dialysis.	Urea, creatinine

ESR=erythrocyte sedimentation rate; MI=myocardial infarction.

REFERENCES

1. Imazio N, Demichelis B, Parrini I, Giuggia M, Cecchi E, Gaschino G, et al. Day-hospital treatment of acute pericarditis: a management program for outpatient therapy. *J Am Coll Cardiol* 2004;**43**:1042–6.
2. Verdona F, Herziga L, Burnandb B, Bischoffa T, Pecoudc A, Junoda M. Chest pain in daily practice:occurrence, causes and management. The TOPIC study. *Swiss Med Weekly* 2008;**138**:240–7.
3. Lange RA, Hillis LD. Acute pericarditis. *N Engl J Med* 2004;**351**:2195–202.
4. Spodick DH. Diagnostic electrocardiographic sequences in acute pericarditis: significance of PR segment and PR vector changes. *Circulation* 1973;**48**:575–80.
5. Imazio M, Cecchi E, Demichelis B, Ierna S, Demarie D, Ghisio A, et al. Indicators of poor prognosis of acute pericarditis. *Circulation* 2007;**115**:2739–44.
6. Adler Y, Charron P, Imazio M, Badano L, Barón-Esquivias G, Bogaert J, et al; ESC Scientific Document Group. 2015 ESC guidelines for the diagnosis and management of pericardial diseases: the task force on the diagnosis and management of pericardial diseases of the European Society of Cardiology (ESC) endorsed by: the European Association for Cardio-Thoracic surgery (EACTS). *Eur Heart J* 2015;**36**(42):2921–64.
7. Imazio M, Brucato A, Cemin R, Ferrua S, Maggiolini S, Beqaraj F, et al; ICAP Investigators. A randomized trial of colchicine for acute pericarditis. *N Engl J Med* 2013;**369**:1522–8.
8. Imazio M, Brucato A, Cemin R, Ferrua S, Belli R, Maestroni S, et al; CORP (Colchicine for Recurrent Pericarditis) Investigators. Colchicine for recurrent pericarditis (CORP): a randomized trial. *Ann Intern Med* 2011;**155**(7):409–14.

CHAPTER 10

Cardiac Biomarker Troponin in Clinical Medicine

CASE 12 SCENARIO: LAURA WITH TROPONIN ELEVATION

Laura is a 42-year-old woman admitted 3 days ago to the intensive care unit following an episode of severe headache and collapse due to a subarachnoid haemorrhage. She is intubated and ventilated. Her routine ECG shows ST-segment depression, T-wave inversion and U waves. Her QT segment is also prolonged.

She is febrile and the initial blood culture shows Gram-positive cocci. She is hypotensive. Her troponin level is 0.6 ng/mL (whereas the normal value is 0.04 ng/mL).

She has no history of ischaemic heart disease. She is a non-smoker. She has no traditional risk factors for ischaemic heart disease. Her bedside echocardiography showed normal left ventricular systolic function without any segmental wall motion abnormalities.

Question

Which of the following statements regarding troponin is true?
1. *A positive result always indicates AMI.*
2. *It has 100% sensitivity and specificity for a diagnosis of AMI.*
3. *The elevation is seen in almost any form of myocardial injury.*
4. *A negative result excludes AMI.*

INTRODUCTION

- Troponin (cTn) is a highly sensitive biomarker of myocardial injury and has been used extensively in everyday clinical practice in the community, as well as in hospitals for the diagnosis of AMI, and for risk stratification of patients with acute coronary symptoms.
- The fourth universal definition of the myocardial infarction consensus document; developed jointly by the European Society of Cardiology, the American College of Cardiology, the American Heart Association, and the World Heart Federation in 2018, issued new criteria that defined the presence of troponin values above the 99th percentile of the upper reference limit as myocardial injury. Occurrence of acute myocardial injury in the setting of acute myocardial ischaemia defines AMI.[1]
- Unfortunately, although the troponin assay is impressively sensitive at detecting cardiac injury, it lacks specificity for diagnosing AMI.

- A large number of clinical conditions other than AMI have now been identified that are associated with a rise in troponin levels.
- Patients who may appear to have no significant cardiac symptoms clinically can present doctors with a diagnostic dilemma. The incorrect diagnosis of MI in patients comes at a significant cost; it often results in further excessive testing and may have medicolegal ramifications as well as effects on patients' health insurance and fitness to drive or work.
- In addition, a wrong diagnosis of MI in a patient based purely on an elevated troponin may result in clinicians missing the true cause of the troponin rise, which can include serious conditions such as pulmonary embolism, sepsis, heart failure, renal failure, pericarditis, etc.[2,3]

HISTOLOGY OF CARDIAC MYOCYTES AND TROPONIN COMPLEX

- Cardiac myocytes contain a basic contractile unit known as a myofibril. Each myofibril is composed of a thick and a thin filament. The troponin complex, actin and tropomyosin combine to form the thin filament, whereas the thick filament is composed of myosin.
- Troponins are cardiac regulatory proteins that control the calcium-mediated interaction of actin and myosin. Upon binding calcium, structural changes occur throughout the actin–tropomyosin filaments to cause muscle contraction.
- The troponin complex itself consists of three subunits: troponin C, I and T.[4,5] Troponin I (cTnI) is uniquely expressed in cardiac muscle[6] and, therefore, assays detecting troponin I are specific for cardiac injury (but not necessarily specific to MI).
- Cardiac troponin C is identical to its skeletal isoform and therefore is not used in a clinical setting to detect cardiac injury, as it is not cardiac specific. Monoclonal antibodies are able to differentiate cardiac troponin T (cTnT) from its skeletal isoform without cross-reactivity; therefore the newer cardiac troponin T assay is now considered equivalent in specificity to assays for cTnI.

MECHANISM OF TROPONIN RELEASE

- Following myocardial injury, troponins are released from the damaged tissue.[7,8] Troponins are known to exist in two pools within myocardial tissue; around 6%–8% of intracellular cardiac troponin T exists in the cytoplasm of cells[7] and as a result is released

immediately, at the time of injury. It is this troponin pool that gives rise to peak serum concentrations within 24–36 hours after injury.[7] However, although troponins have a half-life of approximately 2 hours, in many cases their levels remain elevated in the serum for up to 7–10 days. This is because in irreversible injury there is also a gradual breakdown of myofibrillary-bound complexes from the structural pool as troponin is released from actin during cell death.[7] This results in the characteristic second, blunted peak of serum troponin 2–4 days after myocardial injury. Hence, sustained elevations in troponins are the result of irreversible damage to the structure of the myocardium, whereas transient elevations in troponin levels result from myocardial injuries which are reversible and do not involve myofibrillary breakdowns.

- A transient troponin rise is seen in the setting of sepsis, as well as in experimental models of vital exhaustion and in some exercise studies, which further supports the suggestion that transient troponin elevations originate from reversible injuries which cause a leak from the cytoplasmic troponin pool.[9,10]
- Measuring circulating troponin using highly sensitive assays has become the gold standard approach in diagnosing AMI. However, troponin elevation is found not only in acute coronary syndrome but also in several other conditions (Table 10.1).

TYPE I VS TYPE II MYOCARDIAL INFARCTION

- Troponin elevation is specific for myocardial injury, but not every troponin elevation is due to an MI.
- Type I MI, commonly known as spontaneous MI, is often related to atherosclerotic plaque rupture or erosion, whereas type 2 MI results from MI secondary to ischaemia due to either increased oxygen demand or decreased oxygen supply.[1] Some common causes of type 2 MI include coronary artery spasm, coronary embolism, anaemia, arrhythmia, hypertension and hypotension.
- In the presence of another concurrent acute illness (e.g. sepsis, stroke), differentiation between type I and type 2 MI can be quite challenging and often a more holistic assessment is required. Treatment of type II MI is to treat the underlying condition and hence minimise the cardiac injury.

Troponin in Sepsis and Septic Shock

- Elevation of cardiac troponins is observed in 31%–85% of patients in the setting of sepsis or septic shock. A

TABLE 10.1
Non-Ischaemic Causes and Mechanisms of Troponin Elevation

Underlying Condition	Mechanisms of Troponin Elevation	Comment
Sepsis	Inflammatory cytokine: TNF-alpha, IL-6 Hypotension Tachycardia Noradrenaline/adrenaline Coagulation of capillary bed	High incidence of abnormal cTnI levels in patients with sepsis (31%–85%), most in the absence of CAD on angiography Some correlation of levels with the presence of LV dysfunction by echocardiography and a lower survival rate
Pulmonary embolism	Acute right ventricular strain secondary to increase in pulmonary artery resistance Hypoxaemia Hypoperfusion as a consequence of low output and reduced coronary blood flow	Associated with poor prognosis and increased level predict in-hospital adverse events (death, thrombolysis, CPR, IV catecholamine)
Renal failure	Underlying mechanism is controversial	Elevated value commonly associated with increased all-cause mortality as well as cardiovascular mortality Dynamic changes in troponin values of ≥20% over 6–9 h should be used to define acute MI in ESRD patients
Heart failure	Apoptosis Myocyte damage from neurohormonal activation, inflammatory cytokines Associated coronary artery disease Subendocardial ischaemia	There may be a dose–response relationship between the magnitude of circulating troponin and outcomes Poor diagnostic markers for an ischaemic versus non-ischaemic aetiology of heart failure
Pericarditis	The inflammatory process of acute pericarditis may involve epicardium and cause myocardial damage	Not considered to be a negative prognostic marker
Stroke/intracranial bleed	Activation of the sympathoadrenal system leading to exaggerated catecholamine release and subsequent myocyte injury	Increased troponin level seen in 10% of patients with acute ischaemic stroke and may be higher in haemorrhagic stroke Strong association with inpatient mortality
Takotsubo cardiomyopathy	Catecholamine-induced myocardial stunning	Common presentation includes chest pain in postmenopausal females following emotional stress May show ST elevation in the precordial leads
Tachycardia	Shortening of diastole with subsequent subendocardial ischaemia	In SVT, 48% had elevated troponin
Following angioplasty	Associated with procedural complication such as side-branch occlusion and thrombus formation	Troponin elevation after coronary angioplasty is relatively common
Following endurance exercise	Troponin release most likely due to degradation of 'cytosolic' troponin or increased permeability of myocyte cell membranes under stress	The proportion of individuals with increased troponin concentration following endurance exercise varies widely between studies Increase is typically transient

TABLE 10.1 Non-Ischaemic Causes and Mechanisms of Troponin Elevation—cont'd		
Underlying Condition	**Mechanisms of Troponin Elevation**	**Comment**
Cardiac contusion	Direct damage to the myocytes	Troponins may be elevated after chest wall trauma Increased level may serve to identify patients at increased risk of mortality
Chemotherapy-associated	Mechanism of troponin elevation may include ischaemia, cardiomyopathy and pericarditis	Troponin appears to be a useful tool in detecting chemotherapy-associated cardiac toxicity and stratifying risk for the severity of ventricular dysfunction

CAD=coronary artery disease; CPR=cardiopulmonary resuscitation; ESRD=end-stage renal disease; IL=interleukin; LV=left ventricle; MI=myocardial infarction; SVT=supraventricular tachycardia; TNF=tumour necrosis factor.
(Reproduced with permission, Rahman A, Broadley SA. Elevated troponin: diagnostic gold or fool's gold? *Emerg Med Australas* 2014;26:125–30.)

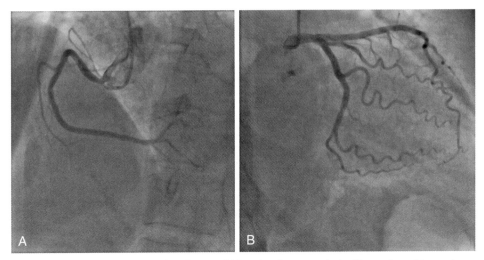

FIG. 10.1 Coronary angiography of a 48-year-old female who presented with sepsis and troponin elevation of 450 ng/L (reference limit <15 ng/L) shows normal epicardial coronary arteries.

majority of patients in this setting have no prior history of coronary artery disease (Fig. 10.1). In these patients there is some correlation between troponin levels and the presence of left ventricular dysfunction as measured by echocardiography, as well as a higher requirement for inotropic medications and a lower survival rate.[11]

- Different theories have been hypothesised to explain the cause of troponin elevation in the setting of sepsis. Most theories suggest that troponin elevation in these instances is multifactorial and results from some level of mismatch between myocardial supply and demand (type 2 MI).

- It has also been suggested that inflammatory cytokines released from neutrophils, particularly tumour necrosis factor alpha (TNF-alpha) and interleukin 6 (IL-6), are responsible for direct myocardial depression and increases in cell membrane permeability to troponin molecules in septic patients.

- In addition, in the setting of sepsis, there is often decreased myocardial perfusion due to hypotension and increased oxygen consumption by cardiac myocytes due to tachycardia. These autonomic responses, as well as the release of noradrenaline and adrenaline, the subsequent vasoconstriction and increased coagulation in the capillary bed could all result in myocyte damage and may contribute to the consequent troponin release in this context.

Troponin Elevation in Pulmonary Embolism

- Pulmonary embolism (PE) shares a number of common symptoms with MI and at times can present with similar ECG changes. Serum troponins are also elevated in up to 50% of patients with PE.[12]
- Troponin elevation in acute PE is thought to result from the increased mechanical load on the right ventricle due to high pulmonary vascular resistance. This results in right ventricular dysfunction and impaired coronary flow superimposed on the hypoxic state caused by the PE.[13]
- A positive troponin test is an important prognostic marker in PE and is more strongly associated with the severity and prognosis of disease than with the diagnosis itself.
- An elevated troponin in the context of PE predicts right ventricular dilation as well as an increased number of segmental perfusion defects on lung scintigraphy.[14] Troponin-positive patients are at increased risk of complications including in-hospital death, prolonged hypotension and cardiogenic shock, and are more likely to require inotropic support and mechanical ventilation. Moreover, an increased troponin value is an independent predictor of 30-day mortality in PE. It is suggested that troponin levels may be used to help risk stratify patients with PE who warrant more aggressive treatment.
- PE has been reported as the most common non-acute coronary syndrome cause of troponin elevation.[15] Whilst CT pulmonary angiography is the gold standard for diagnosis of PE, in the setting of an acute troponin rise, clinicians may be able to differentiate between MI and PE by closely examining the history, looking for the typical ECG findings of PE (Table 10.2) and looking for echocardiographic evidence of right ventricular dysfunction, dilation and increased right ventricular systolic pressures (RVSP).

Troponin Elevation in Renal Failure

- Cardiac troponins are frequently elevated in the absence of acute coronary syndrome among patients with varying degrees of kidney disease; cTnT is more frequently increased than cTnI in asymptomatic patients with end-stage renal disease (ESRD).[16]
- The presence of typical symptoms of ischaemia, ECG changes and cardiac imaging should be used in making the diagnosis of AMI in patients with chronic kidney disease (CKD).

TABLE 10.2
ECG Changes in Stroke

UNDERLYING CARDIAC CONDITION: COMMON RISK FACTORS	RELATED PREEXISTING ECG CHANGES
1. Hypertensive heart disease	1. High QRS voltage; ST, T-wave changes
2. Ischaemic heart disease	2. Pathological Q wave; ST, T-wave changes
3. Arrhythmias	3. Atrial fibrillation/flutter (embolic)

NEW ECG CHANGES FOLLOWING STROKE

1. QT prolongation – most frequent single ECG abnormalities and the most common new ECG finding. Prolongation occurs more frequently following subarachnoid haemorrhage.
2. ST-segment depression and T-wave inversion.
3. U waves.
4. Combinations of QT prolongation, U waves and T-wave changes. Occurs in 8% of stroke patients. Considered 'Classic' changes.

- A survey of non-dialysis ESRD patients reported that serum cTnT was increased above the 99th percentile in 43%, compared with 18% for cTnI. In addition, serum cTnT and cTnI appeared to be increased proportionally with worsening renal function. The exact mechanism underlying increases in cTnT concentrations in patients with kidney disease are not clear. There is emerging evidence that increases in cTnT in asymptomatic patients with ESRD indicate subclinical myocardial necrosis or injury.[17] In addition, cTnT has been found to be a powerful prognostic marker in the ESRD population.[18]
- The NACB Laboratory Medicine Practice Guidelines recommend the use of troponin for diagnosis of MI in all chronic kidney disease patients (regardless of the severity of renal impairment) who have symptoms or electrocardiographic evidence of myocardial ischaemia. In patients with ESRD who have a baseline elevation of cTn and present with signs and symptoms of MI, a dynamic change – defined as an increase in troponin value of at least 20% in the 6–9 hours after presentation – should be considered diagnostic of an acute MI.[19]

Troponin Elevation in Heart Failure

- Troponin elevation in patients with heart failure is relatively common. In the ADHERE (Acute Decompensated Heart Failure National Registry) study, 75%

of patients hospitalised with acute heart failure ($n=67,924$) had detectable levels of cTn (cTnI 0.4 ng/mL or cTnT 0.01 ng/L).[20]

- The mechanism of underlying troponin release in patients with heart failure is not clear and, again, likely to be multifactorial. Although ischaemia is an important cause of heart failure, many patients in heart failure with troponin elevation do not have underlying obstructive coronary artery disease. Proposed mechanisms include subendocardial ischaemia, myocyte damage from inflammatory cytokines, oxidative stress and apoptosis. In addition, it is possible that troponin is being released from viable myocardium as a result of increased permeability of the plasma membrane and leakage of the cytosolic pool of troponin.[21-24]

- Troponin levels may be elevated both in acute and in chronic heart failure. Generally, the magnitude of the troponin elevation is higher in acute heart failure. Numerous studies have demonstrated the association between elevated troponin and adverse clinical outcomes in patients with heart failure, including a markedly increased in-hospital mortality.[20,25] There appears to be a dose–response relationship between the magnitude of circulating troponin and outcomes.

- A meta-analysis involving 16 studies of troponin levels in patients with chronic heart failure revealed that troponin levels predict all-cause and cardiovascular mortality, as well as adverse cardiovascular outcomes.[25]

- Although elevated troponins have prognostic value in heart failure, they are poor diagnostic markers for an ischaemic versus non-ischaemic aetiology of heart failure.

Troponin in Pericarditis

- Serum troponin is reported to be elevated in 32%–49% of cases of acute pericarditis, as a consequence of the involvement of the epicardium in the inflammatory process.[26] Further, ST-segment elevation is more common in troponin I-positive (93%) compared with troponin I-negative (57%) patients. The strong association between troponin release and ST elevation in the setting of pericarditis suggests that troponin release in these patients may be indicative of a more extensive, severe or acute infection which extends to the myocardium, known as myopericarditis.[27] However, in these patients, the underlying pathology or infection type is more closely linked with prognosis than with the presence of a troponin leak.

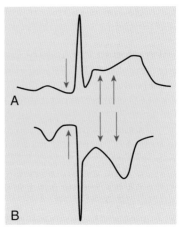

FIG. 10.2 Electrocardiogram changes of: **(A)** diffuse ST-segment elevation (double arrows) and PR-segment depression (single arrow); **(B)** reciprocal PR-segment elevation (single arrow) and ST-segment depression (double arrows) in aVR and occasionally V1. (Reproduced with permission: Rahman A, Liu D. Pericarditis, clinical features and management. *Aust Fam Physician*, 2011;40(10):791–6.)

- Pericarditis often presents with sharp retrosternal pain that may or may not radiate to the neck, shoulder or arms. The pain is often worse when the patient is supine and improves when the patient sits upright or leans forwards. It may be aggravated by deep breathing, swallowing or coughing.

- The pericardial friction rub is the most important physical sign of acute pericarditis.

- ECG changes of widespread ST-segment elevation (in more than one vascular territory) without reciprocal ST depression and/or PR depression (Fig. 10.2) may help distinguish pericarditis from AMI.[28]

- Acute pericarditis is generally diagnosed with at least two of the following criteria: typical chest pain as described above, a pericardial friction rub, suggestive changes on the ECG and a new or enlarging pericardial effusion.

Troponin Elevation in Stroke

- There is a complex overlap between cardiovascular and cerebrovascular disease. Patients with stroke may be prone to MI because of shared risk factors. Left ventricular dysfunction and certain arrhythmias associated with MI are common sources of peripheral embolism or stroke (Box 10.1).

- The cause of troponin rise in acute stroke is not clear. The suggested underlying mechanisms of acute cTn

---

BOX 10.1
ECG Changes in Pulmonary Embolism (PE)

- ECG alone has limited diagnostic utility in the diagnosis of pulmonary embolism and most changes are non-specific.
- ECG findings in acute PE vary depending on the burden of emboli, the degree of pulmonary artery occlusion and level of right ventricular dilation/dysfunction.
- Most of the patients with pulmonary embolism have an abnormality in the ECG. Often the ECG changes simulating myocardial infarction pattern are seen in both inferior and septal leads:
  - Sinus tachycardia is the most common ECG abnormality of pulmonary embolism
  - S1Q3T3 pattern (prominent S wave in lead I, Q wave and inverted T wave in lead III), which occurs in 12%–50% of people with the diagnosis
  - Rightward shift of the QRS axis
  - Atrial fibrillation
  - Transient, complete/incomplete right bundle branch block
  - ST elevation/T-wave inversion in inferior/septal leads.

---

elevation after a stroke include type 1 MI (spontaneous MI, related to atherosclerotic plaque rupture) or type 2 MI (MI secondary to ischaemia due to either increased oxygen demand or decreased supply). It has also been proposed that some of the myocardial damage observed in acute stroke is due to activation of the sympathoadrenal system, leading to exaggerated catecholamine release (probably originating in the right insular cortex) and subsequent myocyte injury.[29]

- Increases in cTn have been reported in all types of stroke, even after patients with ischaemic cardiac damage have been excluded.[30] Increased troponin levels are reported to occur in 5%–34% of patients with acute ischaemic stroke.[31] In several studies, the elevation of troponin in stroke patients provided strong prognostic information about short- and long-term functional outcomes and mortality.[32,33]
- A hospital-based, prospective, observational, case–control study found that elevated serum troponin T was seen in 11% of patients with stroke and was associated with more-severe strokes, larger lesion volumes and a worse outcome. The majority (92%) of patients with elevated serum troponin levels had

anterior circulation infarcts involving the frontal, parietal and insular regions.[33]

Takotsubo Cardiomyopathy and Troponin

- Takotsubo cardiomyopathy (TTC) is a transient form of regional contractile dysfunction with hypokinesia or akinesia of the left ventricle. It is often observed in postmenopausal women where catecholamine-induced vasospasm plays an important role.[34] TTC frequently presents with acute onset of chest pain, electrocardiographic changes and elevated cardiac biomarkers (troponin) in the absence of obstructive coronary artery disease. (See Chapter 11.)
- Unlike AMI, most patients with TTC have a small, rapid increase in troponin levels.[35] Although some studies report a 100% incidence of troponin elevation, the absence of elevation does not exclude the diagnosis of TTC.
- Most patients have a return to normal left ventricular systolic function over 1–4 weeks. They are still, however, at risk of the usual complications of MI until then.
- MRI scanning has shown permanent fibrotic changes in the majority of patients despite their apparently normal left ventricular function.

TACHYARRHYTHMIA

The most likely mechanism for troponin elevation following tachycardia is the shortening of diastole with subsequent subendocardial ischaemia.[36] In a study of 104 patients with a diagnosis of supraventricular tachycardia, elevated serum troponin was seen in 48% of patients.[37]

OTHER CAUSES OF TROPONIN ELEVATION

Troponin elevations have been reported in patients with snake or scorpion bites and these are thought to be due to toxin-mediated myocardial injury, vasospasm and coagulation abnormalities.[38] Elevated cTn levels also have been reported to be elevated frequently in asymptomatic athletes who complete ultra-endurance exercise competitions. The exact mechanism by which cTn release occurs in this setting remains unknown but may be due to right ventricular injury.[39]

Laura made a gradual recovery and was discharged to the rehabilitation unit 12 days later. A myocardial perfusion scan showed 'no reversible perfusion defect'.

Due to its lack of specificity for diagnosing AMI and yet its great sensitivity in detecting myocyte damage, troponin should be considered a biochemical marker that cannot replace the ECG or clinical assessment. Troponin elevations must be interpreted in the clinical context and thus a troponin assay should be performed only if symptoms or history are indicative of MI. Irrespective of the underlying pathology, a troponin elevation is usually indicative of a worse prognosis.

IMPACT OF NEW HIGHLY SENSITIVE TROPONIN ASSAYS IN CLINICAL DECISION MAKING

- Several studies have reported enhanced diagnostic and prognostic accuracy in newly developed, highly sensitive troponin assays across a spectrum of patients with cardiovascular disease.[40]
- High-sensitivity assays allow for earlier detection and risk stratification compared with conventional assays, thus improving triaging and response times in the emergency department. Unfortunately, this improved sensitivity is accompanied by a reduced specificity for the diagnosis of MI compared with standard assays (90.2% vs 97.2%), with positive predictive value as low as 50% in one study.[41]
- In addition, the use of these assays may cause difficulty, as absolute values obtained from different laboratory assays cannot be compared. The high-sensitivity assays are also presented in different units (ng/L, rather than the previous mg/L); 40 ng/L is equivalent to the earlier assay report of 0.04 mg/L.

REFERENCES

1. Thygesen K, Alpert JS, Jaffe AS, Chaitman BR, Bax JJ, Morrow DA, et al; Executive Group on behalf of the Joint European Society of Cardiology (ESC)/American College of Cardiology (ACC)/American Heart Association (AHA)/World Heart Federation (WHF) Task Force for the Universal Definition of Myocardial Infarction. Fourth universal definition of myocardial infarction (2018). *Glob Heart* 2018;**13**(4):305–38.
2. Babuin L, Jaffe AS. Troponin: the biomarker of choice for the detection of cardiac injury. *CMAJ* 2005;**173**:1191–202.
3. Newby LK, Jesse RL, Babb JD, Christenson RH, De Fer TM, Diamond GA, et al. ACCF 2012 expert consensus document on practical clinical considerations in the interpretation of troponin elevations: a report of the American College of Cardiology Foundation task force on Clinical Expert Consensus Documents. *J Am Coll Cardiol* 2012;**60**:2427–63.
4. Takeda S, Yamashita A, Maeda K, Maéda Y. Structure of the core domain of human cardiac troponin in the Ca(2+)-saturated form. *Nature* 2003;**424**:35–41.
5. Schreier T, Kedes L, Gahlmann R. Cloning, structural analysis, and expression of the human slow twitch skeletal muscle/cardiac troponin C gene. *J Biol Chem* 1990;**265**:21247–53.
6. Toyota N, Shimada Y. Differentiation of troponin in cardiac and skeletal muscles in chicken embryos as studied by immunofluorescence microscopy. *J Cell Biol* 1981;**91**:497–504.
7. Katus HG, Remppis A, Scheffold T, Diederich KW, Kuebler W. Intracellular compartmentation of cardiac troponin T and its release kinetics in patients with reperfused and nonreperfused myocardial infarction. *Am J Cardiol* 1991;**67**:1360–7.
8. Maynard SJ, Mentown IBA, Adgey AA. Troponin T or troponin I as cardiac markers in ischaemic heart disease. *Heart* 2000;**83**:3713.
9. Chen Y, Serfass RC, Mackey-Bojack SM, Kelly KL, Titus JL, Apple FS. Cardiac troponin T alterations in myocardium and serum of rats after stressful, prolonged intense exercise. *J Appl Physiol* 2000;**88**:1749–55.
10. Neumayr G, Gaenzer H, Pfister R, Sturm W, Schwarzacher SP, Eibl G, et al. Plasma levels of cardiac troponin I after prolonged strenuous endurance exercise. *Am J Cardiol* 2001;**87**:369–71, A10.
11. Wu AHB. Increased troponin in patients with sepsis and septic shock: myocardial necrosis or reversible myocardial depression? *Intensive Care Med* 2001;**27**:959–61.
12. Goldhaber SZ. Cardiac biomarkers in pulmonary embolism. *Chest* 2003;**123**:1782–4.
13. Giannitsis E, Muller-Bardorff M, Kurowski V, Weidtmann B, Wiegand U, Kampmann M, et al. Independent prognostic value of cardiac troponin T in patients with confirmed pulmonary embolism. *Circulation* 2000;**102**:211–17.
14. Meyer T, Binder L, Hruska N, Luthe H, Buchwald AB. Cardiac troponin I elevation in acute pulmonary embolism is associated with right ventricular dysfunction. *J Am Coll Cardiol* 2000;**36**:632.
15. Ilva T, Eskola M, Nikus K, Voipio-Pulkki L, Lund J, Pulkki K, et al. The etiology and prognostic significance of all-cause troponin I positivity in emergency department patients. *J Emerg Med* 2010;**38**(1):1–5.
16. Apple FS, Murakami MM, Pearce LA, Herzog CA. Predictive value of cardiac troponin I and T for subsequent death in end-stage renal disease. *Circulation* 2002;**106**:2941–5.
17. Ooi DS, Isotalo PA, Veinot JP. Correlation of antemortem serum creatine kinase, creatine kinase-MB, troponin I, and troponin T with cardiac pathology. *Clin Chem* 2000;**46**:338–44.
18. Dierkes J, Domrose U, Westphal S, Ambrosch A, Bosselmann HP, Neumann KH, et al. Cardiac troponin T predicts mortality in patients with end-stage renal disease. *Circulation* 2000;**102**:1964–9.
19. NACB Writing Group, Wu AH, Jaffe AS, Apple FS, Jesse RL, Francis GL, et al. National Academy of Clinical Biochemistry laboratory medicine practice guidelines: use of cardiac troponin and B-type natriuretic peptide or N-terminal proB-type natriuretic peptide for etiologies other than acute coronary syndromes and heart failure. *Clin Chem* 2007;**53**:2086–96.

20. Peacock WF 4th, De Marco T, Fonarow GC, Diercks D, Wynne J, Apple FS, et al. Cardiac troponin and outcome in acute heart failure. *N Engl J Med* 2008;**358**:2117–26.

21. Levine B, Kalman J, Mayer L, Fillit HM, Packer M. Elevated circulating levels of tumor necrosis factor in severe chronic heart failure. *N Engl J Med* 1990;**323**:236–41.

22. Narula J, Haider N, Virmani R, DiSalvo TG, Kolodgie FD, Hajjar RJ, et al. Apoptosis in myocytes in end-stage heart failure. *N Engl J Med* 1996;**335**:1182–9.

23. Olivetti G, Abbi R, Quaini F, Kajstura J, Cheng W, Nitahara JA, et al. Apoptosis in the failing human heart. *N Engl J Med* 1997;**336**:1131–41.

24. Sato Y, Kita T, Takatsu Y, Kimura T. Biochemical markers of myocyte injury in heart failure. *Heart* 2004;**90**:1110–13.

25. Nagarajan V, Hernandez AV, Tang WH. Prognostic value of cardiac troponin in chronic stable heart failure: a systematic review. *Heart* 2012;**98**:1778–86.

26. Brandt RR, Filzmaier K, Hanrath P. Circulating cardiac troponin I in acute pericarditis. *Am J Cardiol* 2001;**87**:1326–8.

27. Newby LK, Ohman EM. Troponins in pericarditis: implications for diagnosis and management of chest pain patients. *Eur Heart J* 2000;**21**:798–800.

28. Spodick DH. Diagnostic electrocardiographic sequences in acute pericarditis: significance of PR segment and PR vector changes. *Circulation* 1973;**48**:575–80.

29. Barber M, Morton JJ, Macfarlane PW, Barlow N, Roditi G, Stott DJ. Elevated troponin levels are associated with sympathoadrenal activation in acute ischaemic stroke. *Cerebrovasc Dis* 2007;**23**:260–6.

30. Sandhu R, Aronow WS, Rajdev A, Sukhija R, Amin H, D'aquila K, et al. Relation of cardiac troponin I levels with in-hospital mortality in patients with ischemic stroke, intracerebral hemorrhage, and subarachnoid hemorrhage. *Am J Cardiol* 2008;**102**:632–4.

31. Kerr G, Ray G, Wu O, Stott DJ, Langhorne P. Elevated troponin after stroke: a systematic review. *Cerebrovasc Dis* 2009;**28**:220–6.

32. Di Angelantonio E, Fiorelli M, Toni D, Sacchetti ML, Lorenzano S, Falcou A, et al. Prognostic significance of admission levels of troponin I in patients with acute ischaemic stroke. *J Neurol Neurosurg Psychiatry* 2005;**76**:76–81.

33. Ghali J, Allison D, Kleinig T, Ooi SY, Bastiampillai S, Ashby D, et al. Elevated serum concentrations of troponin T in acute stroke: what do they mean? *J Clin Neurosci* 2010;**17**(1): 69–73.

34. Rahman A, Liu D. Broken heart syndrome – a case study. *Aust Fam Physician* 2012;**41**:55–8.

35. Ramaraj R, Sorrell V, Movahed MR. Levels of troponin release can aid in the early exclusion of stress-induced (takotsubo) cardiomyopathy. *Exp Clin Cardiol* 2009;**14**:6–8.

36. Jeremias A, Gibson M. Alternative causes for elevated cardiac troponin levels when acute coronary syndromes are excluded. *Ann Intern Med* 2005;**142**:786–91.

37. Bukkapatnam RN, Robinson M, Turnipseed S, Tancredi D, Amsterdam E, Srivatsa UN. Relationship of myocardial ischemia and injury to coronary artery disease in patients with supraventricular tachycardia. *Am J Cardiol* 2010;**106**:374–7.

38. Kelley WE, Januzzi JL, Christenson RH. Increases of cardiac troponin in conditions other than acute coronary syndrome and heart failure. *Clin Chem* 2009;**55**(12):2098–112.

39. Shave R, Baggish A, George K, Wood M, Scharhag J, Whyte G, et al. Exercise-induced cardiac troponin elevation: evidence, mechanisms, and implications. *J Am Coll Cardiol* 2010; **56**(3):169–76.

40. Keller T, Zeller T, Peetz D, Tzikas S, Roth A, Czyz E, et al. Sensitive troponin I assay in early diagnosis of acute myocardial infarction. *N Engl J Med* 2009;**361**:868–77.

41. Morrow DA. Clinical application of sensitive troponin assays. *N Engl J Med* 2009;**361**:913–15.

CHAPTER 11

Takotsubo Cardiomyopathy

KEY POINTS

- Takotsubo cardiomyopathy should be suspected in any postmenopausal woman presenting with chest pain and dyspnoea following intense emotional or physical stress.
- ECG changes are often dramatic and not in proportion with the rise in troponin levels.
- Acute coronary syndrome is an important differential diagnosis and suspected cases should be referred to hospital.
- Generally, the diagnosis can be confirmed by findings of normal coronary arteries and apical ballooning of the left ventricle on coronary angiography.
- Heart failure with or without pulmonary oedema is the most common clinical complication of takotsubo cardiomyopathy.
- The prognosis of takotsubo cardiomyopathy is usually good, with a mortality rate of 0%–8%. Most patients that survive the initial episode regain normal ventricular function within 1–4 weeks.

CASE 13 SCENARIO: EDITH WITH CHEST PAIN AND DYSPNOEA

Edith, 65 years of age, lives in a rural township. She experienced sudden onset severe chest pain and dyspnoea after learning that her husband had died. Edith's daughter drove her to the local hospital where investigations were performed. Investigations included an electrocardiogram (ECG), a blood test for troponin I, chest x-ray (CXR) and echocardiogram.

Edith's ECG is shown in Fig. 11.1; her troponin I was elevated, at 1.1 µg/L (reference range <0.04 µg/L). An urgent mobile CXR revealed no evidence of pneumothorax and a normal mediastinum. A bedside echocardiogram was then organised urgently and this revealed a large anteroseptal and apical area of akinesia (Fig. 11.2). Her calculated LV function was 24%.

Edith had a coronary angiogram performed and that showed normal epicardial coronary arteries (Fig. 11.3) with apical akinesia and hypercontractile basal segments on the ventriculogram (Fig. 11.4) consistent with a diagnosis of takotsubo cardiomyopathy.

The ECG changes shown may have a number of differential diagnoses, and in some cases without clinical correlation, these may be difficult to distinguish. In this case, takotsubo cardiomyopathy (TTC) is the most likely diagnosis.

DIFFERENTIAL DIAGNOSES

- **Acute non-ST elevation myocardial infarction (NSTEMI):** it is not uncommon for a patient with a diagnosis of NSTEMI to present with chest pain, dyspnoea and T-wave inversion on the ECG with troponin elevation. The ECG changes in NSTEMI are confined typically to one vascular territory. In Edith's case, the T-wave inversion is diffuse. This makes the diagnosis of NSTEMI less likely.
- **Acute pulmonary embolism:** patients with pulmonary embolism often present with pleuritic chest pain, dyspnoea, troponin elevation and ECG changes that include sinus tachycardia, S1Q3T3 pattern or changes in the inferior and septal leads. These typical changes are absent in Edith's case.

THE HISTORY OF TAKOTSUBO CARDIOMYOPATHY AND ITS NOMENCLATURE

- Takotsubo cardiomyopathy was first described by Sato and colleagues in 1990.[1] It is described as a depression of the contractile function of the mid and apical segments of the left ventricle, with compensatory hyperkinesis of the basal walls. This leads to ballooning of the ventricular apex during systole.
- It was given the name 'takotsubo' because of the visual similarities with a traditional Japanese

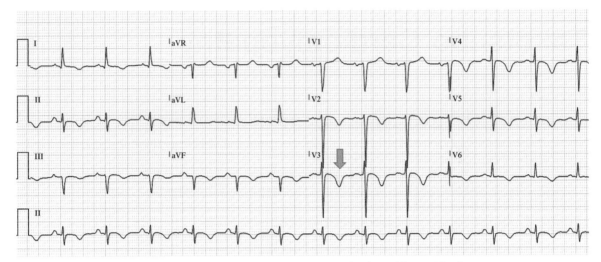

FIG. 11.1 ECG showing deep T-wave inversion (arrow) in most leads.

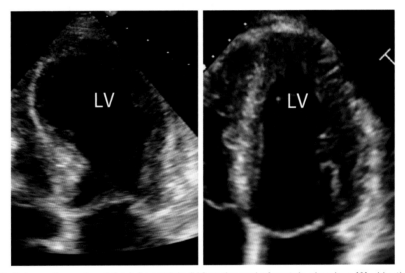

FIG. 11.2 Echocardiography of the left ventricle (LV) at the end of systole showing: **(A)** akinetic, ballooned apex of a patient with takotsubo cardiomyopathy; **(B)** a normal apex.

octopus-catching pot (in Japanese 'takotsubo' means 'fishing pot for trapping octopus').

- Its prevalence has been shown to be 1.2%–2.2% of all patients who present with a suspected acute coronary syndrome.[2]
- As takotsubo cardiomyopathy is usually triggered by physical or emotional stress, the alternative terms 'stress cardiomyopathy' and 'broken heart syndrome' are often used. It has also been called 'apical ballooning syndrome' because of the balloon-like appearance

of the left ventricle during systole on echocardiography or ventriculography.

PATHOGENESIS OF TAKOTSUBO CARDIOMYOPATHY

The most commonly postulated pathogenesis of takotsubo cardiomyopathy is that an intensely stressful emotional or physical trigger causes an excess of circulating catecholamines, which causes both direct

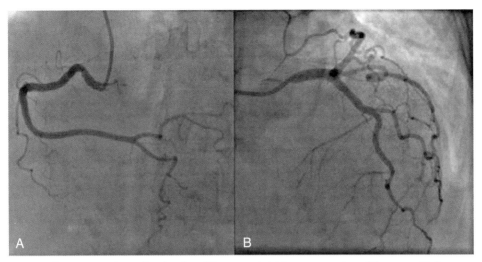

FIG. 11.3 Coronary angiography showing: **(A)** a normal right coronary artery; **(B)** a normal left coronary artery on the right.

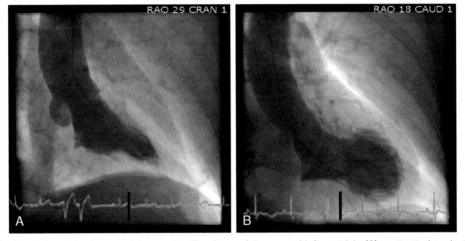

FIG. 11.4 A ventriculogram of the contractile phase of the normal left ventricle **(A)** contrasted against a takotsubo cardiomyopathy ventriculogram showing apical ballooning of the left ventricle **(B)**.

myocardial toxicity and microvascular dysfunction leading to myocardial stunning and consequent contractile dysfunction. The denser distribution of adrenoceptors at the apex might explain why the apex is usually affected whereas the base of the ventricle is spared.[3] Oestrogen downregulates cardiac adrenoceptors and attenuates their response to activation, providing a plausible reason for why the condition is largely confined to postmenopausal women.[4]

PRESENTATION OF TAKOTSUBO CARDIOMYOPATHY

- Takotsubo cardiomyopathy mimics acute coronary syndrome in presentation and is seen most commonly in postmenopausal women following intense emotional or physical stress. Physical triggers (36%) were found to be more common than emotional triggers (27.7%).[5]

- Cases in the literature report a wide range of triggers including an unexpected death in the family, gambling and financial losses, receiving a devastating medical diagnosis, motor vehicle accidents, stress caused from public speaking, acute physical trauma, robbery and major surgical procedures. Sometimes good news can be the trigger (e.g. winning the lottery).[2] However, in approximately 20%–35% of cases no obvious precipitant can be found.[6]
- More than half (55.8%) of patients with takotsubo cardiomyopathy may have a history of a neurological or psychiatric disorder.[5]
- The most common presenting symptom in takotsubo cardiomyopathy is acute chest pain (75.9%). A patient may also present with dyspnoea (46.9%) or syncope (7.7%).[5]

INVESTIGATIONS
ECG Changes in Takotsubo Cardiomyopathy
- The most common acute ECG findings of takotsubo cardiomyopathy are ST-segment elevation in the precordial leads and T-wave inversion in most leads.[7]
- Unlike the picture in acute myocardial infarction, the ECG changes in takotsubo cardiomyopathy are not limited to one coronary vascular territory. This differs from the typical ECG changes in an acute STEMI, which include elevation of the ST segments in contiguous leads accompanied by reciprocal ST depression in leads remote from the site of an acute infarct.
- Characteristic ECG findings in takotsubo cardiomyopathy are shown in Table 11.2. Electrocardiographic changes are often dramatic and out of proportion to the modest changes in troponin levels.
- Electrocardiogram changes that may be seen in pulmonary embolism include sinus tachycardia, complete or incomplete (R) bundle branch block, S1Q3T3 pattern (deep S wave in lead 1, pathological Q wave and T-wave inversion in lead 3) and ST elevation or T-wave inversion in inferior and septal leads.

INVESTIGATIONS INCLUDING CARDIAC ENZYMES IN TAKOTSUBO CARDIOMYOPATHY
- Unlike in the situation in acute myocardial infarction, most patients with takotsubo cardiomyopathy have a small but rapid increase in cardiac enzyme and biomarker levels. Although some series reported a 100% incidence of troponin elevation, the absence of elevation does not exclude the diagnosis of takotsubo cardiomyopathy.
- Recent data from the International Takotsubo Registry showed that troponin levels were elevated in 87% of the patients with a diagnosis of TTC, with a mean level similar to those inpatients with acute coronary syndromes.[5]
- It is suggested that if the levels of troponin T are greater than 6 ng/mL and troponin I are greater than 15 ng/mL, the diagnosis of takotsubo cardiomyopathy is unlikely and an acute coronary syndrome should be considered as the primary diagnosis. Troponin T also shows a significant inverse correlation with the initial ejection fraction.[8] (See Chapter 10.)
- The creatine kinase level is generally not substantially elevated in the majority of patients with takotsubo cardiomyopathy, but 82.9% of patients may have elevated levels of brain natriuretic peptide on admission.[5]

Other Investigations
- Although a CXR may be normal, patients can present with acute pulmonary oedema and cardiomegaly.
- Though the proposed diagnostic criteria for TTC include absence of obstructive coronary disease on coronary angiography, the presence of coronary artery disease does not exclude the diagnosis of TTC. Over 15% of patients with takotsubo cardiomyopathy have evidence of co-existing coronary artery disease on angiography.[5]
- Coronary angiography in the Takotsubo Italian Network registry similarly showed 9.6% patients had at least one relevant (≥50%) stenotic coronary artery not supplying the dysfunctional myocardium.
- It was proposed that when the stenotic artery does not supply the dysfunctional myocardium, or when the extent of dysfunctional myocardium is wider than the territory of distribution supplied by a single stenotic coronary artery, the presence of angiographically relevant CAD should not be considered an exclusion criterion for TTC.[9]
- Cardiac MRI may detect regional wall motion abnormalities of the ventricle that extend beyond a single epicardial vascular distribution. Unlike myocardial infarction, late gadolinium enhancement on cardiac MRI is generally absent in TTC.

CLASSIFICATION OF TAKOTSUBO CARDIOMYOPATHY
Takotsubo cardiomyopathy can be classified into four types depending on the location of the contractile dysfunction (Table 11.1).

PROGNOSIS AND COMPLICATIONS OF TAKOTSUBO CARDIOMYOPATHY

- The prognosis of takotsubo cardiomyopathy has generally been considered good in the past, but recent follow-up of the International Takotsubo Registry showed that 21.8% of patients had a combined end point of serious in-hospital complications with rates equal to or higher than those of patients with an acute coronary syndrome.
- Patients with TTC also had severe complications, including ventricular tachycardia (3%), ventricular thrombus (1.3%) and ventricular rupture (0.2%) (Box 11.1).[10]
- During the 30 days after admission, the rate of major adverse cardiac and cerebrovascular events was 7.1%.
- Long-term follow-up of patients revealed a rate of death from any cause of 5.6% per patient-year and a rate of major adverse cardiac and cerebrovascular events of 9.9% per patient-year.
- The rate of recurrence of TTC was 1.8% per patient year.[5]

TABLE 11.1
Types of Takotsubo Cardiomyopathy Based on Wall Motion Abnormality[3]

Type	Description
Classic, apical ballooning or takotsubo type	Apical ballooning (most commonly reported)
Reverse apical ballooning or reverse takotsubo type	Hyperdynamic apex and akinesia of the base of the left ventricular wall (uncommon)
Midventricular type	Involves the mid left ventricular wall, sparing the base and the apex
Local type	Localised wall motion abnormality affecting a segment of the left ventricular wall; most often affects the anterior wall

TABLE 11.2
Electrocardiogram (ECG) Changes in Takotsubo Cardiomyopathy

ECG Change	Example	Prevalence in TTC
ST-segment elevation, most commonly in precordial leads		Common (46%–100%)
Diffuse deep symmetric T-wave inversion; resolves slowly and often partially		Common
Pathological Q waves that typically resolve before hospital discharge, with restoration of normal R-wave progression		37%
Prolonged Q–T interval, which is 1–2 days		

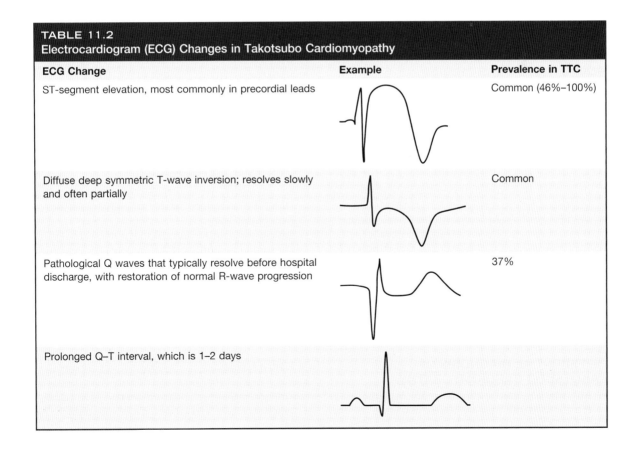

BOX 11.1
Complications of Takotsubo Cardiomyopathy[10]

- Left heart failure with or without pulmonary oedema
- Cardiogenic shock
- Dynamic intraventricular obstruction with left ventricular intracavity pressure gradient generation
- Mitral regurgitation resulting from chordal tethering and systolic anterior motion of the mitral valve apparatus
- Ventricular arrhythmias
- Left ventricular mural thrombus formation
- Left ventricular free wall rupture
- Death

- Patients who survive the acute episode typically recover normal ventricular function within 1–4 weeks. Subtle, persisting fibrotic changes may be seen on MRI scanning, however.
- Heart failure with or without pulmonary oedema is the most common clinical complication and was reported in 38 of 215 patients (17.7%).[11]

PROPOSED DIAGNOSTIC CRITERIA

The proposed 'Mayo Clinic' diagnostic criteria for takotsubo cardiomyopathy include:

- echocardiographic or angiographic evidence of transient hypokinesis, akinesis or dyskinesis of the left ventricle beyond a single epicardial coronary artery perfusion territory
- often, but not always, a stressful trigger
- the absence of obstructive coronary disease or angiographic evidence of acute plaque rupture
- new ECG abnormalities or modest elevation in troponins
- the absence of phaeochromocytoma or myocarditis.[12]

Without the use of coronary angiography, it can be difficult objectively to distinguish takotsubo cardiomyopathy from acute coronary syndrome. When the diagnosis is in doubt, takotsubo cardiomyopathy should be treated as acute coronary syndrome until proven otherwise. Most patients should be hospitalised for confirmation of the diagnosis and subsequent management.

DIFFERENTIAL DIAGNOSIS OF TAKOTSUBO CARDIOMYOPATHY

- An acute coronary syndrome (with or without ST elevation) is the primary differential diagnosis as both disease states have significant overlap in their clinical presentations. Coronary angiography may help to differentiate the two conditions. It is likely to show significant coronary artery disease, or evidence of acute plaque rupture in the coronary artery supplying the dysfunctional ventricular muscle territory, in patients with acute coronary syndrome.
- Other differential diagnoses include: myocarditis, endogenous catecholamine excess (phaeochromocytoma), exogenous catecholamine excess (cocaine, amphetamine), peripartum cardiomyopathy and cerebrovascular disease.
- Differential diagnoses for chest pain such as aortic dissection, pulmonary embolism should also be considered.[13]

MANAGEMENT OF TAKOTSUBO CARDIOMYOPATHY

- Treatment of takotsubo cardiomyopathy is usually supportive. Despite the fact that a beta-blockade is widely considered to have an important role in treatment, there is a lack of large randomised controlled trials to support its routine use. Recent data from the International Takotsubo Registry did not show any benefits of using beta-blockers in the acute phase of TTC. Beta-blockers also did not show any benefits in preventing recurrence of TTC.[5]
- In haemodynamically stable patients, a beta-blocker could be considered in selective cases and diuretics given as necessary for volume overload. Beta-blockers may block the effects of the catecholamine excess, which is a potential mechanism of takotsubo cardiomyopathy. Moreover, beta-blockers have an essential role in reducing left ventricular outflow tract obstruction by decreasing basal-segment hypercontractility.[10]
- In a rodent model, takotsubo cardiomyopathy could be prevented with an alpha-blockade or beta-blockade.[14]
- Patients without a left ventricular outflow tract gradient should be prescribed an angiotensin-converting enzyme (ACE) inhibitor or an angiotensin receptor antagonist to prevent cardiac remodelling. Recent data from the International Takotsubo Registry showed use of angiotensin-converting enzyme inhibitors or angiotensin receptor blockers was associated with improved survival at 1 year.[5]

Edith remained well on day three and was discharged on a small dose of a beta-blocker and ACE inhibitor. Follow-up was arranged with her general practitioner in 7 days and with a cardiology clinic 4 weeks after a repeat echocardiography.

REFERENCES

1. Sato H, Tateishi H, Uchida T, Dote K, Ishihara M, Sasaki K. Tako-tsubo-like left ventricular dysfunction due to multivessel coronary spasm. In: Kodama K, Haze K, Hori M, editors. *Clinical aspect of myocardial injury: from ischemia to heart failure*. Tokyo: Kagakuhyoronsha; 1990. pp. 56–64.
2. Abdulla I, Ward MR. Takotsubo cardiomyopathy: how stress can mimic acute coronary occlusion. *Med J Aust* 2007;**187**:357–60.
3. Tsuchihashi K, Ueshima K, Uchida T, Oh-mura N, Kimura K, Owa M, et al; Angina Pectoris-Myocardial Infarction Investigations in Japan. Transient left ventricular apical ballooning without coronary artery stenosis: a novel heart syndrome mimicking acute myocardial infarction. Angina Angina Pectoris-Myocardial Infarction Investigations in Japan. *J Am Coll Cardiol* 2001;**38**:11–18.
4. Ueyama T, Hano T, Kasamatsu K, Yamamoto K, Tsuruo Y, Nishio I. Estrogen attenuates the emotional stress induced cardiac responses in the animal model of takotsubo (Ampulla) cardiomyopathy. *J Cardiovasc Pharmacol* 2003;**42**(Suppl. 1):S117–19.
5. Templin C, Ghadri JR, Diekmann J, Napp LC, Bataiosu DR, Jaguszewski M, et al. Clinical features and outcomes of takotsubo (stress) cardiomyopathy. *N Engl J Med* 2015;**373**(10):929–38.
6. Abdulla I, Kay S, Mussap C, Nelson GI, Rasmussen HH, Hansen PS, et al. Apical sparing in takotsubo cardiomyopathy. *Intern Med J* 2006;**36**:414–18.
7. Vivo RP, Krim SR, Hodgson J. It's a trap! Clinical similarities and subtle ECG differences between takotsubo cardiomyopathy and myocardial infarction. *J Gen Intern Med* 2008;**23**:1909–13.
8. Ramaraj R, Sorrell VL, Movahed MR. Levels of troponin release can aid in the early exclusion of stress-induced (takotsubo) cardiomyopathy. *Exp Clin Cardiol* 2009;**14**:6–8.
9. Parodi G, Citro R, Bellandi B, Del Pace S, Rigo F, Marrani M, et al; Tako-tsubo Italian Network (TIN). Tako-tsubo cardiomyopathy and coronary artery disease: a possible association. *Coron Artery Dis* 2013;**24**:527–33.
10. Wittstein IS, Thiemann DR, Lima JA, Baughman KL, Schulman SP, Gerstenblith G, et al. Neurohumoral features of myocardial stunning due to sudden emotional stress. *N Engl J Med* 2005;**352**:539–48.
11. Gianni M, Dentali F, Grandi AM, Sumner G, Hiralal R, Lonn E. Apical ballooning syndrome or takotsubo cardiomyopathy: a systematic review. *Eur Heart J* 2006;**27**:1523–9.
12. Bybee KA, Kara T, Prasad A, Lerman A, Barsness GW, Wright RS, et al. Systematic review: transient left ventricular apical ballooning: a syndrome that mimics ST-segment elevation myocardial infarction. *Ann Intern Med* 2004;**141**:858–65.
13. Gopalakrishnan P, Zaidi R, Sardar MR. Takotsubo cardiomyopathy: pathophysiology and role of cardiac biomarkers in differential diagnosis. *World J Cardiol* 2017;**9**(9):723–30.
14. Ueyama T, Kasamatsu K, Hano T, Yamamoto K, Tsuruo Y, Nishio I. Emotional stress induces transient left ventricular hypocontraction in the rat via activation of cardiac adrenoceptors: a possible animal model of 'takotsubo' cardiomyopathy. *Circ J* 2002;**66**:712–13.

CHAPTER 12

Atrial Fibrillation

KEY POINTS

- Atrial fibrillation (AF) is the most common cardiac arrhythmia that typically causes an 'irregularly irregular' pulse.
- A number of other clinical conditions can also cause an irregular pulse.
- Treatment strategy of AF includes: control of the ventricular rate (rate control), rhythm control, minimising the risk of thromboembolism and treatment of the underlying condition.
- Beta-blockers, non-dihydropyridine calcium channel blockers and digoxin are the main drugs used to control the ventricular rate.
- Drugs commonly used for rhythm control strategies are flecainide, amiodarone and sotalol.
- The major risk associated with AF is a cardioembolism stroke, which can be minimised by appropriate use of anticoagulants.
- Oral anticoagulation in the form of vitamin K antagonists (VKAs) is a well-established treatment for stroke prevention in AF.
- New oral anticoagulants are broadly preferable to VKA in the vast majority of patients with non-valvular AF.
- The evidence for effective stroke prevention with aspirin in AF is weak.

CASE 14 SCENARIO: JUNE HAS AN IRREGULAR PULSE

June is a 75-year-old female patient who presents to the general practice surgery with frequent palpitations, weakness, decreased effort tolerance and dyspnoea. Examination reveals an 'irregularly irregular' pulse.

June's medical history includes hypertension and type 2 diabetes. She had a stroke 2 years previously without any residual weakness. She has no history of heart failure, ischaemic heart disease or peripheral arterial disease. June's medications include perindopril 10 mg daily, aspirin 100 mg daily and metformin 500 mg twice daily. Her electrocardiogram (ECG) is shown in Fig. 12.1. Her thyroid function and renal/liver function tests are normal.

Atrial fibrillation is the most common cardiac arrhythmia. It affects more men than women and is more prevalent with increasing age. AF occurs in fewer than 1% of persons aged 60–65 years, but in 8%–10% of those older than 80 years.[1]

- AF is a supraventricular arrhythmia characterised by disorganised atrial activity with associated loss of atrial contraction, a reduction in cardiac output and atrial thrombus formation. This leads to significant complications, the most frequent major complication being a stroke or systemic embolisation. AF

is detected clinically as an irregularly irregular pulse.
- Patients with AF are frequently asymptomatic. Typical symptoms include palpitations, shortness of breath, reduced exercise tolerance, chest pain and tiredness. AF is often recognised during a routine physical examination, on an ECG or during the interrogation of pacemakers placed for bradyarrhythmias in patients with no history of AF.
- An ECG during an episode is the only way to confirm the diagnosis. If the diagnosis is suspected and the ECG is normal, longer monitoring with an external or implanted loop recorder may establish the diagnosis.

DIFFERENTIAL DIAGNOSIS OF AN IRREGULARLY IRREGULAR PULSE
(Table 12.1, Fig. 12.2)
Atrial fibrillation typically causes an irregularly irregular pulse. However, a number of other clinical conditions can also cause an irregular (either regularly irregular or irregularly irregular) pulse, including:
- second-degree heart block
- atrial or ventricular ectopic
- atrial flutter with variable heart block
- sinus arrhythmia (generally causes regularly irregular pulse).

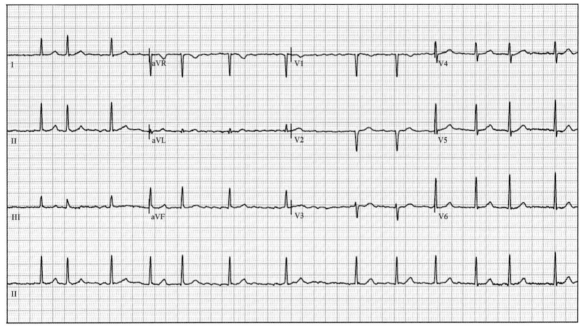

FIG. 12.1 ECG showing absence of P waves and various durations of P–R interval with irregular QRS complex. The P waves are replaced by fibrillatory f waves.

TABLE 12.1
Irregular Pulse

Conditions	ECG Features	Clinical Importance
Atrial fibrillation	• Absence of P waves • Fibrillatory waves • Variable ventricular rate	• Relatively common • Increased risk of stroke and systemic embolism • Risk of tachycardia-induced cardiomyopathy when ventricular rate is poorly controlled
Atrial flutter	• 'Sawtooth' flutter waves with regular atrial activities • When associated with variable block, it is associated with irregular ventricular response	• Like atrial fibrillation, atrial flutter is associated with an increased risk stroke and systemic embolism
Second-degree heart block	• Mobitz type I (Wenckebach phenomenon) – progressive prolongation of the P–R interval, with eventual non-conducted P wave • Mobitz II – intermittent non-conducted P waves; the P–R interval in the conducted beats remains constant	• Mobitz I is usually a benign rhythm; asymptomatic patients do not require treatment. • Patients with Mobitz II heart block may require permanent pacemaker insertion
Atrial ectopic	• An abnormal P wave followed by QRS complex; typically, a P wave has a different morphology	• Atrial ectopic are generally benign arrhythmias
Ventricular ectopic	• Wide QRS complex (>120 ms) with compensatory pause	• Patient often presents with symptoms of 'skipping a beat' • Generally benign
Sinus arrhythmia	• Cyclical lengthening and shortening of P–R interval with respiration	• It is a normal physiological phenomenon and is often present in young, healthy individuals

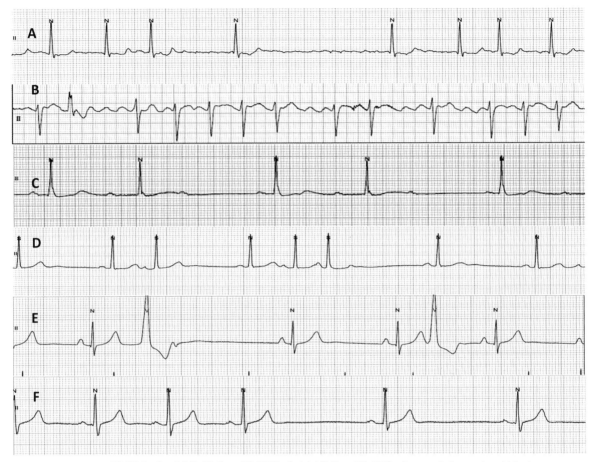

FIG. 12.2 **(A)** ECG of atrial fibrillation. **(B)** ECG of atrial flutter. **(C)** ECG of second-degree heart block, Mobitz I. **(D)** ECG of atrial ectopics/premature atrial complexes. **(E)** ECG of ventricular ectopics/ventricular premature contractions. **(F)** ECG of sinus arrhythmia.

Some of the conditions are relatively benign, whereas other conditions are not. An ECG is very important in order to establish the diagnosis. In AF, there is typically an absence of P waves and irregularly irregular QRS complexes.

CLASSIFICATION OF ATRIAL FIBRILLATION

The classification of AF is shown in Table 12.2.

THE TREATMENT STRATEGY OF ATRIAL FIBRILLATION[2]

The treatment strategy includes:
- control of the ventricular rate (rate control)
- achievement and maintenance of sinus rhythm (rhythm control)

TABLE 12.2
Classification of Atrial Fibrillation (AF)[2]

Paroxysmal AF	AF that terminates spontaneously or with intervention within 7 days of onset
Persistent AF	Continuous AF that is sustained >7 days
Long-standing persistent AF	Continuous AF lasting for ≤1 year
Permanent AF	Permanent AF means that the arrhythmia is continuous, and interventions to restore sinus rhythm have either failed or a rhythm control strategy is not considered any more

- minimising the risk of thromboembolism
- treatment of underlying conditions.

Control of the Ventricular Rate (Rate Control)

- Pharmacological agents commonly used to control ventricular rates in AF are beta-blockers (e.g. metoprolol, atenolol), non-dihydropyridine calcium channel blockers (e.g. diltiazem, verapamil) or digoxin (Table 12.3).[3,4]
- Intravenous amiodarone can be useful for rate control in selected patients.
- Atrioventricular (AV) nodal ablation with permanent ventricular pacing is reasonable to control heart rate when pharmacological therapy is inadequate, the patient experiences unacceptable side effects to medications or when rhythm control is not achievable.

Achievement and Maintenance of Sinus Rhythm (Rhythm Control)[5]

- Rhythm control involves conversion to normal sinus rhythm with electrical direct current cardioversion (DCCV) or with antiarrhythmic drugs (see Table 12.3).
- Compared with rate control, rhythm control generally does not improve mortality, the frequency of a stroke, hospitalisation or quality of life.
- The AFFIRM (Atrial Fibrillation Follow-up Investigation of Rhythm Management) trial, has shown there is no difference in survival between the 'rate control' and 'rhythm control' strategy. There is also no significant difference between the two groups in the rates of the secondary end point of death, disabling stroke, major bleeding or cardiac arrest. There were more adverse drug effects in the rhythm control group compared with the rate control group.[6]

TABLE 12.3
Common Drugs/Methods Used for Atrial Fibrillation (AF) in Australia

Drugs	Uses	Important Considerations
DRUGS USED IN RATE CONTROL		
Beta-blockers	• Beta-blocker monotherapy is often the first-line rate-controlling agent • Improvement in both resting and exercise rate control for beta-blockers	• Contraindicated in asthma • Most common adverse symptoms are lethargy, dizziness, bradycardia
Non-dihydropyridine calcium channel blockers	• Diltiazem or verapamil is effective in reducing ventricular rate both at rest and during exercise	• Should be avoided in patients with reduced ejection fraction because of their negative inotropic effects
Digoxin	• Digoxin can be used to slow ventricular heart rate • Digoxin is effective only for ventricular rate control at rest • Digoxin has the advantage of slowing the ventricular rate without lowering the blood pressure • Digoxin has no effect on mortality in heart failure patients with reduced ejection fraction in sinus rhythm but reduces hospital admissions[3]	• Not very effective in hyperadrenergic patients • Dosage adjustment is required in renal impairment • Digoxin is not useful for conversion of AF to sinus rhythm
Amiodarone	• IV amiodarone can be useful in selected patients for rate control when other agents have failed or are contraindicated • Steady state of drug may not be established for several months • Has class I, II, III, IV antiarrhythmic action	• IV amiodarone can cause significant bradycardia • Can have a number of extra cardiac side effects including thyroid problems, pulmonary toxicity
Direct current cardioversion (DCCV)	• Electrical cardioversion could be considered in haemodynamically unstable patient with rapid ventricular rate	• Duration of AF needs to be considered before DCCV • AF >48 hours (or unknown duration), transoesophageal ECG-guided cardioversion may be considered

TABLE 12.3
Common Drugs/Methods Used for Atrial Fibrillation (AF) in Australia—cont'd

Drugs	Uses	Important Considerations
DRUGS USED IN RHYTHM CONTROL		
Flecainide	• Flecainide is the best agent for pharmacological cardioversion of AF, unless contraindicated • Can be self-administered by the patient at home to restore sinus rhythm after safety has been established in the hospital setting • Flecainide does not usually alter the heart rate and should be co-administered with BB, verapamil, digoxin	• Should not be used in presence of structural heart disease, second- or third-degree AV block, post-MI and significant renal or hepatic impairment • Bioavailability 95% • Peak plasma level 2–4 h • Half-life 12–27 h[4]
Amiodarone	• Amiodarone best agent for long-term maintenance of sinus rhythm • It also slows the ventricular response at rest and with exercise. and may reduce symptoms associated with rapid ventricular response to AF • Can at times result in pharmacological cardioversion of AF and precautions need to be taken to prevent thromboembolic events • The risk of thromboembolic events does not differ between electrical and pharmacological conversion	• Amiodarone safe from cardiac point of view but significant non-cardiac side effect • 2% incidents of pulmonary fibrosis • 6% hypothyroidism, 0.9% hyperthyroidism • Neuropathy in 0.6%/year • Elevated liver enzymes 10%–20%[4] • Amiodarone can be used in patients with heart failure and in patients with ischaemic heart disease
Sotalol	• Helpful for rate control as well as for rhythm control	• Need to adjust dose in patients with renal insufficiency
Dronedarone	• Dronedarone is a multichannel-blocking drug similar in structure to amiodarone but without iodine	• Contraindicated in patients with decompensated heart failure
Electrical cardioversion	• Immediate efficacy of DCCV exceeds 90%	• In AF for >48 hours duration, anticoagulation for at least 3 weeks before and 4 weeks after cardioversion is recommended

AV=atrioventricular; BB=beta-blocker; MI=myocardial infarction.

- Similarly, in patients with AF and congestive heart failure (EF <35%), a routine strategy of rhythm control does not reduce the rate of death from cardiovascular causes, as compared with a rate-control strategy.[7]
- A rhythm control strategy may be useful in symptomatic patients and in younger patients without structural heart disease.
- Drugs commonly used for termination of AF and maintenance of sinus rhythm (rhythm control strategy) are flecainide, amiodarone and sotalol.

Electrical cardioversion
- Electrical cardioversion (ECV) is indicated when the patient is haemodynamically unstable, when drugs are ineffective or contraindicated and when the duration of AF is prolonged.

- For patients who have been in AF for longer than 48 hours, or when the duration of AF is unknown, oral anticoagulants should be started at least 3 weeks before cardioversion and continued for at least 4 weeks afterwards.
- When warfarin is used, the target international normalised ratio (INR) should be achieved between 2 and 3 for at least 3 weeks before cardioversion.
- Non-vitamin-K antagonist oral anticoagulants (NOACs) have been increasingly used as an alternative to warfarin before elective cardioversion. The anticoagulant effect of NOACs fades rapidly 12–24 h after the last intake and strict therapy compliance by the patient is crucial for adequate protection. If compliance with NOAC intake can be reliably confirmed, cardioversion seems acceptably safe.[8]

- For NOAC patients in whom low compliance is suspected despite proper education and additional tools, conversion to warfarin could be considered.
- As an alternative to anticoagulation prior to cardioversion, transoesophageal echocardiography (TOE) guided cardioversion can be used to confirm the absence of a thrombus within the left atrium.

Catheter ablation of atrial fibrillation

- Catheter ablation of AF is effective in restoring and maintaining sinus rhythm in selective patients with paroxysmal or persistent AF who are symptomatic, refractory or intolerant to antiarrhythmic drug therapy. Most patients require more than one procedure to achieve symptom control.
- Five to seven percent of patients suffer from severe complications after catheter ablation of AF, and 2%–3% experience life-threatening complications. The most important severe complications of catheter ablation are a stroke, cardiac tamponade, pulmonary vein stenosis and atrio-oesophageal fistula.[9]

Minimising the Risk of Thromboembolism

- The major risk associated with AF is ischaemic stroke, frequently occurring from a cardioembolism source (Fig. 12.3). Factors that predispose to stroke include increasing age, history of previous stroke or transient ischaemic attack (TIA), hypertension, diabetes, congestive cardiac failure and current smoking. Other factors include female sex and vascular disease. Previously unknown AF is associated with about 10% of all ischaemic strokes.

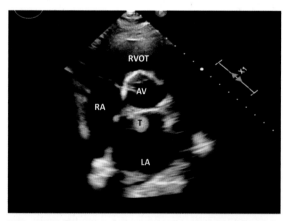

FIG. 12.3 Parasternal short-axis view showing left atrial thrombus in a patient with atrial fibrillation. AV=aortic valve; LA=left atrium.; RA=right atrium; RVOT=right ventricular outflow tract; T=thrombus.

- Oral anticoagulation (OAC) can prevent the majority of ischaemic strokes in AF patients and can prolong life. It is superior to no treatment or aspirin in patients with different profiles for stroke risk. The net clinical benefit is almost universal, with the exception of patients at very low stroke risk, and OAC should therefore be used in most patients with AF.[10]
- Oral anticoagulation in the form of vitamin K antagonists (VKAs) is a well-established treatment for stroke prevention in AF. VKAs (warfarin) have also been used extensively over the past 50 years in the treatment and prevention of deep venous thrombosis and pulmonary embolism, and for the prevention of thromboembolism in mechanical valves.[2,11]

Vitamin K antagonists (warfarin) and non-vitamin-K antagonist oral anticoagulants

- The NOACs currently approved in Australia are dabigatran, rivaroxaban and apixaban. The NOACs can be classified into the direct thrombin inhibitors (dabigatran) and factor Xa inhibitors: rivaroxaban, apixaban and edoxaban.
- Edoxaban (30 or 60 mg once daily), approved in 2015 by the US Food and Drug Administration (FDA), was studied in a large randomised prospective AF trial; it was found to be non-inferior to warfarin with regard to the prevention of stroke or systemic embolisation, and was associated with significantly lower rates of bleeding and death from cardiovascular causes.[12]
- The NOACs so far tested in clinical trials have all shown non-inferiority when compared with VKAs, as well as better safety, consistently reducing the number of intracranial haemorrhages.[13]
- The major positive aspects of NOACs over VKAs are that:
  - they do not require regular INR monitoring
  - there is reduced risk of adverse interactions with concomitant use of other drugs or changes in the diet
  - they are effective for prevention of strokes
  - effective antidotes have become available for one of the agents.[14]
- On this basis, the 2012 focused update of the European Society of Cardiology guidelines[15] for the management of AF recommends NOACs as 'broadly preferable to VKA in the vast majority of patients with non-valvular AF'.
- The term 'valvular AF' indicates that AF is related to rheumatic valvular disease (predominantly moderate to severe mitral stenosis) or the presence of mechanical heart valves. All the major trials involving NOACs excluded patients with valvular AF. Generally, warfarin

TABLE 12.4
The CHADS2 and CHADS2DS2-VASc scores[17]

A. CHADS2 VS CHADS2DS2-VASC SCORE

CHADS2 Score			CHA2DS2-VASc Score		
C	Congestive heart failure	1 point	C	Congestive heart failure	1 point
H	Hypertension	1 point	H	Hypertension	1 point
A	Age >75 years	1 point	A2	Age >75 years	2 points
D	Diabetes	1 point	D	Diabetes	1 point
S2	Stroke	2 points	S2	Stroke	2 points
			V	Vascular disease	1 point
			A	Age> 65 years	1 point

B. ADJUSTED RISK OF STROKE FOR CHADS2 AND CHA2DS2–VASC SCORES

Score	CHADS2 (%/Year)	CHA2DS2–VASc (%/Year)
0	1.9	0
1	2.8	1.3
2	4	2.2
3	5.9	3.2
4	8.5	4
5	12.5	6.7
6	18.2	9.8
7		9.6
8		6.7
9		15.2

is the preferred treatment option in that clinical setting.

- Stable patients taking warfarin whose INR is within the targeted therapeutic range, and in whom INR testing does not present a problem, may prefer to continue with warfarin.
- In the absence of head-to-head trials, it is inappropriate to be definitive about which of the NOACs is best, given the heterogeneity of the different trials. There is insufficient evidence to recommend one NOAC over another, although some patient characteristics, drug compliance and tolerability, drug interaction and cost may be important considerations in the choice of agents.[16]
- Though there is a lack of head-to-head trials, dabigatran 110 mg BD and apixaban 2.5 mg twice daily seem to have a slightly lower bleeding risk profile.[15]
- The current limitations of NOACS are: limited availability of the effective antidote, increased risk of bleeding (albeit less than warfarin), inability to

determine patients' compliance, dose adjustment in renally and hepatically impaired patients, increased cost compared with warfarin.

Current indications for NOACs[15,16]

- Prevention of stroke in patients with non-valvular AF (except with moderate-to-severe mitral stenosis or a mechanical heart valve) with a CHA2DS-2VASc/CHADS2 score of 2 in males and 3 in females (see Table 12.4).[17]
- Prophylaxis of deep vein thrombosis/pulmonary embolism in patients undergoing knee or hip replacement surgery.
- Treatment of deep vein thrombosis/pulmonary embolism.

Important landmark NOACs trials. Important landmark trials have shown all NOACs to be at least non-inferior to VKAs, with less major bleeding risk in patients with non-valvular AF.

- In the Rocket AF trial, rivaroxaban was found to be non-inferior to warfarin for the prevention of stroke and thromboembolism. This trial enrolled 14,264 patients who were randomised to either rivaroxaban or warfarin. The risk of major bleeding in the rivaroxaban group was no different compared with the warfarin group, while intracranial haemorrhage (0.5% versus 0.7%, P=0.02) and fatal bleeding (0.2% versus 0.5%, P=0.003) were reduced.[18]
- Apixaban was evaluated against warfarin in the ARISTOTLE trial, in which 18,201 patients were enrolled. Apixaban was superior to warfarin in preventing stroke or systemic embolisation, while causing less bleeding and mortality.[19]
- Dabigatran was compared with warfarin in the RELY trial in which 18,113 patients were enrolled. Dabigatran at a dose of 110 mg was associated with rates of stroke and systemic embolism that were similar to those associated with warfarin (1.53% versus 1.69%, P<0.001), as well as lower rates of major haemorrhage (2.71% per year in the group receiving 110 mg dabigatran compared with 3.36% per year in the group receiving warfarin; P=0.003).[20]
- A meta-analysis of randomised trials showed NOACs had a favourable risk–benefit profile, with significant reduction in stroke, intracranial haemorrhage and mortality, and with similar major bleeding as warfarin, but increased gastrointestinal bleeding.[21]

Measurement of anticoagulant effect
- Dabigatran: the activated partial thromboplastin time (aPTT) may provide a qualitative assessment of dabigatran level and activity; if the aPTT level at trough (19–31) is double the upper limit of normal, this may be associated with a higher risk of bleeding.[22]
- Dabigatran has also little effect on INR and prothrombin time (PT).
- Rivaroxaban and apixaban: PT and aPTT are affected to a varying extent by the Xa inhibitors; aPTT cannot be used for any meaningful evaluation of Xa inhibitory effect.[23]
- Importantly, INR is completely unreliable in monitoring the anticoagulant effect of the factor Xa inhibitors. If INR is elevated, it may be a marker of vitamin K deficiency that needs to be separately corrected.

CHADS2 vs CHADS2-VASc score[24,25]. There are different stroke risk stratification schemes to optimise antithrombotic/anticoagulant treatment.
- For patients with non-valvular AF (the term 'valvular AF' is used to imply that AF is related to rheumatic valvular disease, predominantly mitral stenosis and prosthetic heart valves), the CHADS2 score is a commonly used, validated, clinical prediction score that uses congestive heart failure, hypertension, age >75 years, diabetes and history of stroke or TIA in a cumulative manner to estimate expected stroke rate per 100 patient years (Table 12.4).
- Unfortunately, the CHADS2 score has limitations and does not include many common potential stroke risk factors such as female sex and left ventricular ejection fraction.[26]
- Therefore, new guidelines developed by the European Society of Cardiology recommend a risk factor-based approach with a new schema: the CHA2DS2-VASc score (see Table 12.4).
- The CHA2DS2-VASc schema places greater emphasis on major risk factors, including age >75 years and previous episodes of stroke/TIA, by allocating two points to each, with one point for the presence of each of the other clinically relevant non-major risk factors.
- The CHA2DS2-VASc score improves risk prediction and is better at identifying 'truly low-risk' patients with AF. Table 12.4 shows the adjusted risk of stroke for CHADS2 and CHA2DS2-VASc scores. For patients with AF and an elevated CHA2DS2-VASc score of 2 or greater in men or 3 or greater in women, oral anticoagulants are recommended.[16]

Factors that need to be considered before starting a NOAC[27]
- Before starting a NOAC, one of the most important considerations should be the renal function. Most of the NOACs are contraindicated if there is significant renal impairment (estimated glomerular filtration rate (eGFR) <30 mL/min). If there is moderate renal impairment, NOACs could be used with caution and, in most cases, dosages need to be reduced.
- A meta-analysis of patients with mild-to-moderate renal impairment (eGFR >30 mL/min) found that NOACs, including direct thrombin inhibitors and Factor Xa inhibitors, were superior to warfarin. They also have better safety profiles, with less risk of major bleeding.[28]
- For patients with AF who have a CHA2DS2-VASc score of 2 or greater in men or 3 or greater in women and who have end-stage chronic kidney disease (CKD) (creatinine clearance (CrCl) <15 mL/min) or are on dialysis, it might be reasonable to prescribe warfarin (INR 2.0 to 3.0) or apixaban for oral anticoagulation.[17]

- NOACs are not recommended for use in patients with severe hepatic dysfunction.
- Compliance and adherence to treatment are crucial, especially as these drugs have a relatively short half-life.

Antiplatelet agents as an alternative to an anticoagulant

- Aspirin is often considered in patients who either are not candidates for anticoagulation (e.g. patients with increased bleeding risk) or are low-risk patients on the basis of a CHADS2/CHA2DS2-VASc score. Unfortunately, the evidence for effective stroke prevention with aspirin in AF is weak and should be limited to the few patients who refuse any form of oral anticoagulants.[15]
- A meta-analysis confirmed that warfarin, which is considered the standard therapy, is superior to single and combination antiplatelet therapy in the prevention of stroke. Adjusted doses of warfarin and aspirin reduce the risk of stroke by 64% and 22%, respectively. In the ACTIVE-W trial, warfarin therapy reduced the rate of stroke by 42% compared with therapy with clopidogrel plus aspirin.[29]
- Data indicate that the risk of major bleeding or intracranial haemorrhage with aspirin is not significantly different to that of oral anticoagulants, especially in the elderly.[30]
- The 2018 National Heart Foundation of Australia and Cardiac Society of Australia and New Zealand guidelines for the diagnosis and management of AF do not recommend antiplatelet therapy for stroke prevention, regardless of stroke risk.[31]

Management of patients with atrial fibrillation and coronary artery disease

- There is significant overlap between AF and coronary artery disease. Patients with a history of AF taking an anticoagulant requiring elective stenting, or presenting with acute coronary syndrome, frequently require antiplatelet agents. The composition and duration of antiplatelet agents and anticoagulant depend on careful balancing of the risk of thrombosis and the risk of bleeding.
- In a patient with AF presenting for an elective angioplasty due to coronary disease, current guidelines recommend 1 month of triple therapy, generally with either a reduced dose of oral anticoagulant (15 mg of rivaroxaban daily, 110 mg twice-daily dabigatran or 2.5 mg twice-daily apixaban) in combination with aspirin and clopidogrel, followed by dual therapy (an oral anticoagulant plus a single antiplatelet agent,

either aspirin or clopidogrel) for up to 6–12 months depending on bleeding risk, with continuation of oral anticoagulant monotherapy thereafter.
- For angioplasty in the setting of an acute coronary syndrome, the ESC guidelines[10] recommend between 1 month and 6 months of triple therapy in the high-bleeding-risk and low-bleeding-risk groups (HAS-BLED score above 3 or between 0 and 2) respectively, followed by dual therapy for the remainder of the 12-month period.

Double therapy vs triple therapy

- Although 'triple therapy' offers the best protection against thrombosis, it also increases the risk of bleeding significantly. A number of recent trials recently showed that 'double therapy' with an oral anticoagulant and single antiplatelet agent reduces risk of bleeding significantly but, unfortunately, none of the trials clearly gives us the answer as to whether the risk of thrombosis is increased with the omission of aspirin.
- An open-label, multicentre, randomised controlled trial, assessing the use of clopidogrel with or without aspirin in patients taking oral anticoagulant therapy (warfarin) and undergoing percutaneous coronary intervention, found that the use of clopidogrel without aspirin is associated with a significant reduction in bleeding complications and no increase in the rate of thrombotic events.[32]

Left atrial appendage occlusion[17,33]

- Percutaneous left atrial appendage occlusion may be considered for stroke prevention in selected patients with AF who are unable to tolerate anticoagulants due to serious life-threatening bleeding.
- A Watchman device (a percutaneous left atrial appendage occlusion device as an alternative to anticoagulant), when compared with warfarin therapy in randomised trials, has been found to be non-inferior to warfarin treatment in the prevention of stroke in AF patients with moderate stroke risk, with a possibility of lower bleeding rates. Unfortunately, the implantation procedure can be associated with significant, life-threatening risk of complications.

Assessing bleeding risk

Decision-making for prophylaxis of thromboembolism needs to balance the risk of stroke against the risk of major bleeding. The NOACs offer an alternative to warfarin therapy for selected patients, but, as with all anticoagulants, they can potentially cause serious bleeding.

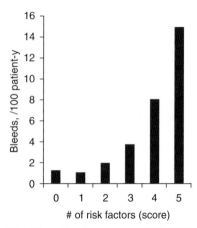

Letter	Clinical Characteristic	Points Awarded
H	Hypertension	1
A	Abnormal renal and liver function (1 point each)	1 or 2
S	Stroke	1
B	Bleeding	1
L	Labile INRs	1
E	Elderly (e.g. age >65 years)	1
D	Drugs or alcohol (1 point each)	1 or 2
		Maximum 9 points

FIG. 12.4 Bleeding risk: the HAS-BLED score. The HAS-BLED score can be used to evaluate major bleeding risk in patients with AF taking warfarin or NOAC therapy. (From Pisters R, Lane DA, Nieuwlaat R, de Vos CB, Crijns HJ, Lip GY. A novel user-friendly score (HAS-BLED) to assess 1-year risk of major bleeding in patients with atrial fibrillation: The Euro Heart Survey. *Chest* 2010;138:1093–100; Belen E, Canbolat IP, Bayyigit A, Helvaci A, Pusuroglu H, Kilickesmez K. A new gap in the novel anticoagulants' era: undertreatment. *Blood Coagul Fibrinolysis* 2015;26:793–7; ESC Guidelines. Guidelines for the management of atrial fibrillation: The Task Force for the management of atrial fibrillation of the European Society of Cardiology (ESC). 2010. *Eur Heart J* 2010;31:2369–429, with permission of Oxford University Press.)

The HAS-BLED score (Fig. 12.4) was developed as a practical risk score to estimate the 1-year risk for major bleeding in patients with AF.[34]

The HAS-BLED score gives 1 point each for the presence of:
- hypertension (systolic blood pressure >160 mmHg)
- abnormal renal or liver function (1 point each):
  - abnormal renal function (dialysis, transplant, creatinine >2.26 mg/dL or >200 mmol/L).
  - abnormal liver function (cirrhosis or bilirubin twice the upper limit of normal and aspartate aminotransferase (AST), alanine aminotransferase (ALT) and alkaline phosphatase (ALP) three times the upper limit of normal)
- history of stroke or TIA
- prior major bleeding or predisposition to bleeding
- labile INRs (i.e. unstable/high INRs, time in therapeutic anticoagulation of <60%)
- age over 65 years
- drug or alcohol use (1 point each):
  - more than eight standard drinks (alcohol) per week
  - use of drugs predisposing to bleeding such as non-steroidal anti-inflammatory drugs (NSAIDs), antiplatelet agents.

A HAS-BLED score of 3 and above means that regular clinical review to monitor bleeding is recommended following the initiation of anticoagulant therapy.

Treatment of Underlying Conditions

- A full medical history and physical examination should be performed to explore symptoms and signs of thyrotoxicosis, structural heart disease, and heart failure, and treated appropriately.
- Basic blood tests, including a thyroid function test, should be performed to exclude thyrotoxicosis as the underlying cause of AF. Serum electrolytes and renal and liver function tests should be performed to guide the selection of drug therapy, and stool examination considered for occult blood before starting anticoagulation.
- Transthoracic echocardiography is useful to exclude underlying structural heart disease that may not otherwise be recognised and can identify tachycardia-induced cardiomyopathy, which may occur when in fibrillation with an inadequately controlled ventricular rate for an extended period. Eighty percent of patients with AF have some form of structural heart disease, particularly hypertensive heart disease, coronary artery disease, valvular heart disease or cardiomyopathy (Fig. 12.5).[2]
- In selected cases when clinical suspicion is high, an additional test to exclude pulmonary embolism may be indicated. If the patient has a history of unusual tiredness, or snoring, they may need to have a formal sleep study to exclude obstructive sleep apnoea.

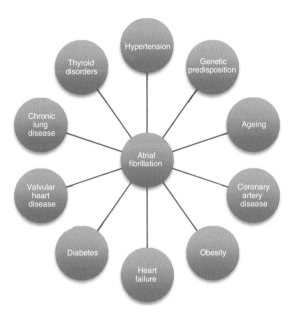

FIG. 12.5 Aetiology of atrial fibrillation.

June was prescribed with rivaroxaban 20 mg once daily owing to her preference for once-daily dosage.

REFERENCES

1. Kannel WB, Benjamin EJ. Current perceptions of the epidemiology of atrial fibrillation. *Cardiol Clin* 2009;**27**:13–24.

2. January CT, Wann LS, Alpert JS, Calkins H, Cigarroa JE, Cleveland JC Jr, et al; American College of Cardiology/American Heart Association Task Force on Practice Guidelines. 2014 AHA/ACC/HRS guideline for the management of patients with atrial fibrillation: a report of the American College of Cardiology/American Heart Association Task Force on Practice Guidelines and the Heart Rhythm Society. *J Am Coll Cardiol* 2014;**64**(21):e1–76.

3. The Digitalis Investigation Group. The effect of digoxin on mortality and morbidity in patients with heart failure. *N Engl J Med* 1997;**336**:525–33.

4. Opie LH, Gersh BJ. *Drugs for the heart*. 8th ed. Philadelphia: Elsevier Saunders; 2013.

5. de Denus S, Sanoski CA, Carlsson J, Opolski G, Spinler SA. Rate vs rhythm control in patients with atrial fibrillation: a meta-analysis. *Arch Intern Med* 2005;**165**:258–62.

6. Wyse DG, Waldo AL, DiMarco JP, Domanski MJ, Rosenberg Y, Schron EB, et al. Atrial Fibrillation Follow-up Investigation of Rhythm Management (AFFIRM) Investigators. A comparison of rate control and rhythm control in patients with atrial fibrillation. *N Engl J Med* 2002;**347**:1825–33.

7. Roy D, Talajic M, Nattel S, Wyse DG, Dorian P, Lee KL, et al. Atrial Fibrillation and Congestive Heart Failure Investigators. Rhythm control versus rate control for atrial fibrillation and heart failure. *N Engl J Med* 2008;**358**:2667–77.

8. Cappato R, Ezekowitz MD, Klein AL, Camm AJ, Ma CS, Le Heuzey JY, et al. Rivaroxaban vs. vitamin K antagonists for cardioversion in atrial fibrillation. *Eur Heart J* 2014;**35**(47):3346–55.

9. Dagres N, Hindricks G, Kottkamp H, Sommer P, Gaspar T, Bode K, et al. Complications of atrial fibrillation ablation in a high-volume center in 1,000 procedures: still cause for concern? *J Cardiovasc Electrophysiol* 2009;**20**:1014–19.

10. Kirchhof P, Benussi S, Kotecha D, Ahlsson A, Atar D, Casadei B, ESC Scientific Document Group. 2016 ESC Guidelines for the management of atrial fibrillation developed in collaboration with EACTS. *Eur Heart J* 2016;**37**:2893–962.

11. Australian Government Department of Health. *Pharmaceutical Benefits Scheme information*. Woden, ACT: DoH; 2020. www.pbs.gov.au.

12. Giugliano RP, Ruff CT, Braunwald E, Murphy SA, Wiviott SD, Halperin JL, et al; ENGAGE AF-TIMI 48 Investigators. Edoxaban versus warfarin in patients with atrial fibrillation. *N Engl J Med* 2013;**369**:2093–104.

13. Ruff CT, Giugliano RP, Braunwald E, Hoffman EB, Deenadayalu N, Ezekowitz MD, et al. Comparison of the efficacy and safety of new oral anticoagulants with warfarin in patients with atrial fibrillation: a meta-analysis of randomised trials. *Lancet* 2014;**383**:955–62.

14. Wadhera RK, Russell CE, Piazza G. Cardiology patient page. Warfarin versus novel oral anticoagulants: how to choose? *Circulation* 2014;**130**(22):e191–3.

15. Camm AJ, Lip GY, De Caterina R, Savelieva I, Atar D, Hohnloser SH, et al. ESC Committee for Practice Guidelines (CPG). 2012 focused update of the ESC Guidelines for the management of atrial fibrillation: an update of the 2010 ESC Guidelines for the management of atrial fibrillation. Developed with the special contribution of the European Heart Rhythm Association. *Eur Heart J* 2012;**33**(21):2719–47.

16. January CT, Wann LS, Calkins H, Chen LY, Cigarroa JE, Cleveland JC Jr, et al. 2019 AHA/ACC/HRS focused update of the 2014 AHA/ACC/HRS guideline for the management of patients with atrial fibrillation: a report of the American College of Cardiology/American Heart Association Task Force on Clinical Practice Guidelines and the Heart Rhythm Society. *J Am Coll Cardiol* 2019;**74**(1):104–32.

17. Pison L, Potpara TS, Chen J, Larsen TB, Bongiorni MG, Blomstrom-Lundqvist C. Left atrial appendage closure-indications, techniques, and outcomes: results of the European Heart Rhythm Association Survey. *Europace* 2015;**17**:642–6.

18. Patel MR, Mahaffey KW, Garg J, Pan G, Singer DE, Hacke W, et al. ROCKET AF Investigators. Rivaroxaban versus warfarin in nonvalvular atrial fibrillation. *N Engl J Med* 2011;**365**(10):883–91.

19. Granger CB, Alexander JH, McMurray JJ, Lopes RD, Hylek EM, Hanna M, et al. ARISTOTLE Committees and Investigators. Apixaban versus warfarin in patients with atrial fibrillation. *N Engl J Med* 2011;**365**(11):981–92.

20. Healey JS, Eikelboom J, Douketis J, Wallentin L, Oldgren J, Yang S, et al; RE-LY Investigators. Periprocedural bleeding and thromboembolic events with dabigatran compared to warfarin: results from the RE-LY randomized trial. *Circulation* 2012;**126**(3):343–8.

21. Ruff CT, Giugliano RP, Braunwald E, Hoffman EB, Deenadayalu N, Ezekowitz MD, et al. Comparison of the efficacy and safety of new oral anticoagulants with warfarin in patients with atrial fibrillation: a meta-analysis of randomised trials. *Lancet* 2014;**383**:955–62.

22. Van Ryn J, Stangier J, Haertter S, Liesenfeld KH, Wienen W, Feuring M, et al. Dabigatran etexilate – a novel, reversible, oral direct thrombin inhibitor: interpretation of coagulation assays and reversal of anticoagulant activity. *Thromb Haemost* 2010;**103**:1116–27.

23. Lindhoff-Last E, Samama MM, Ortel TL, Weitz JI, Spiro TE. Assays for measuring rivaroxaban: their suitability and limitations. *Ther Drug Monit* 2010;**32**:673–9.

24. Gage BF, Waterman AD, Shannon W, Boechler M, Rich MW, Radford MJ. Validation of clinical classification schemes for predicting stroke: results from the National Registry of Atrial Fibrillation. *JAMA* 2001;**285**:2864–70.

25. Lip GYH, Nieuwlaat R, Pisters R, Lane DA, Crijns HJ. Refining clinical risk stratification for predicting stroke and thromboembolism in atrial fibrillation using a novel risk factor based approach: the Euro Heart survey on atrial fibrillation. *Chest* 2010;**137**:263–72.

26. Karthikeyan G, Eikelboom JW. The CHADS2 score for stroke risk stratification in atrial fibrillation – friend or foe? *Thromb Haemost* 2010;**104**:45–8.

27. Heidbuchel H, Verhamme P, Alings M, Antz M, Diener HC, Hacke W, et al. Updated European Heart Rhythm Association Practical Guide on the use of non-vitamin K antagonist anticoagulants in patients with non-valvular atrial fibrillation. *Europace* 2015;**17**(10):1467–507.

28. De-Caprio Munoz F, Gharacholou SM, Munger TM, Friedman PA, Asirvatham SJ, Packer DL, et al. Meta-analysis of renal function on the safety and efficacy of novel oral anticoagulants for atrial fibrillation. *Am J Cardiol* 2016;**117**(1):69–75.

29. ACTIVE Writing Group of the ACTIVE Investigators, Connolly S, Pogue J, Hart R, Pfeffer M, Hohnloser S, et al. Clopidogrel plus aspirin versus oral anticoagulation for atrial fibrillation in the Atrial fibrillation Clopidogrel Trial with Irbesartan for prevention of Vascular Events (ACTIVE W): a randomised controlled trial. *Lancet* 2006;**367**(9526):1903–12.

30. Mant J, Hobbs FD, Fletcher K, Roalfe A, Fitzmaurice D, Lip GY, et al; BAFTA investigators; Midland Research Practices Network (MidReC). Warfarin vs. aspirin for stroke prevention in an elderly community population with atrial fibrillation (the Birmingham Atrial Fibrillation Treatment of the Aged Study, BAFTA): a randomised controlled trial. *Lancet* 2007;**370**:493–503.

31. NHFA CSANZ Atrial Fibrillation Guideline Working Group, Brieger D, Amerena J, Attia J, Bajorek B, Chan KH, et al. National Heart Foundation of Australia and the Cardiac Society of Australia and New Zealand: Australian clinical guidelines for the diagnosis and management of atrial fibrillation 2018. *Heart Lung Circ* 2018;**27**(10):1209–66.

32. Dewilde WJ, Oirbans T, Verheugt FW, Kelder JC, De Smet BJ, Herrman JP, et al. WOEST study investigators. Use of clopidogrel with or without aspirin in patients taking oral anticoagulant therapy and undergoing percutaneous coronary intervention: an open-label, randomised, controlled trial. *Lancet* 2013;**381**(9872):1107–15.

33. Reddy VY, Holmes D, Doshi SK, Neuzil P, Kar S. Safety of percutaneous left atrial appendage closure: results from the WATCHMAN Left Atrial Appendage System for embolic protection in patients with AF (PROTECT AF) clinical trial and the Continued Access Registry. *Circulation* 2011;**123**(4):417–24.

34. Pisters R, Lane DA, Nieuwlaat R, de Vos CB, Crijns HJ, Lip GY. A novel user-friendly score (HAS-BLED) to assess 1-year risk of major bleeding in patients with atrial fibrillation: the Euro Heart Survey. *Chest* 2010;**138**:1093–100.

CHAPTER 13

Perioperative Management of Anticoagulants/Antiplatelet Agents

CASE 15 SCENARIO: MR JOHNSON WITH HYPERTENSION AND AF

Mr Johnson is a 72-year-old who presents to the surgery for the removal of a skin lesion on his right forearm. His background medical history includes hypertension, diet-controlled diabetes and persistent atrial fibrillation (AF). He had a stroke 3 years ago without any residual weakness. His medications include perindopril 10 mg daily and rivaroxaban 20 mg daily. ECG shows atrial fibrillation with a ventricular rate of 57 beats per minute.

Questions
1. *Does he need to stop his rivaroxaban prior to the procedure? If so, how soon before?*
2. *When will you consider restarting his anticoagulant after the procedure?*

CASE16 SCENARIO: MR SMITH WITH ANGINA

Mr Smith is a 73-year-old undergoing an excision of cutaneous lesions with simple flap closure. Following episodes of chronic stable angina, he had a stent inserted in the right coronary artery 2 weeks previously. He is on aspirin and clopidogrel.

Questions

1. *Does he need to stop antiplatelet agents prior to surgery?*
2. *How soon prior to the procedure will you stop them?*
3. *How soon can it be restarted after surgery?*

A large number of patients in clinical practice are taking oral anticoagulant or antiplatelet drugs for primary or secondary prevention of arterial or venous thrombosis. There is an increased risk of bleeding when patients take anticoagulant or antiplatelet drugs during surgery. The decision over whether or not to continue the drug during surgery, and when to stop and restart, involves balancing the risks of arterial or venous thrombo-embolism against the risk of bleeding.

Oral anticoagulation in the form of vitamin K antagonists (VKAs) is a well-established treatment for stroke prevention in atrial fibrillation. VKAs have also been used extensively over the past 50 years in the treatment and prevention of deep venous thrombosis, pulmonary embolism and for the prevention of thromboembolism in mechanical valves. While the non-vitamin-K antagonist oral anticoagulants (NOACs) offer an alternative to warfarin therapy for selected patients, like all anticoagulants they are a class of medicines that can potentially cause serious bleeding.

The current Pharmaceutical Benefits Scheme (PBS)-approved indications for NOACs are listed in Box 13.1.[1]

The major positive aspects of these agents include:
- no need for monitoring
- reduced risk of adverse interactions with a change in diet or concomitant drugs
- effective for the prevention of strokes.
  The current limitations of NOACS are:
- the limited availability of an effective antidote
- increased risk of bleeding (albeit less than warfarin)
- inability to determine patients' compliance
- dose adjustment in renally and hepatically impaired patients
- increased cost compared with warfarin.
  In addition to anticoagulants, antiplatelet agents including aspirin, clopidogrel, ticagrelor and prasugrel are widely used in Australia for the treatment and prevention of vascular disease.

Table 13.1 summarises the strategies of perioperative use of the three NOACs available on the PBS (dabigatran, rivaroxaban and apixaban), aspirin, warfarin and common antiplatelet agents (clopidogrel, ticagrelor and prasugrel).

BOX 13.1
Current Indications for Using NOACs

A. Prevention of stroke or systemic embolism in a patient with non-valvular atrial fibrillation who is at moderate-to-high risk of developing stroke or systemic embolism as evidenced by one or more of the following risk factors:
   a. age 75 years or older
   b. hypertension
   c. diabetes mellitus
   d. heart failure or left ventricular dysfunction (ejection fraction less than 40%)
   e. previous stroke or transient ischaemic attack or systemic embolism.

(The term 'valvular atrial fibrillation' is used to imply that AF is related to rheumatic valvular disease (predominantly mitral stenosis) or prosthetic heart valves. Rheumatic mitral valve disease with AF carries a 17-fold increased risk of stroke and requires anticoagulation with warfarin. AF in patients with prosthetic valves also requires anticoagulation with warfarin, usually with a higher INR target dependent on the types of valves.)

B. Prophylaxis of deep vein thrombosis/pulmonary embolism in patients undergoing knee or hip replacement surgery.

C. Treatment of deep vein thrombosis/pulmonary embolism.

ORAL ANTICOAGULANT THERAPY IN THE PERIPROCEDURAL PERIOD

- Surgical interventions or invasive procedures that carry a significant risk of bleeding may require temporary cessation of the NOAC or warfarin (Fig. 13.1). Trials have previously shown that about one in four patients who need anticoagulation therapy require temporary cessation of their anticoagulants within 2 years.[2]
- When the anticoagulants are discontinued in high-risk patients, the interval without anticoagulation should be as short as possible with the risk of thrombo-embolism balanced against the risk of bleeding.

Predicting the Risk of Thrombosis

- For patients with non-valvular atrial fibrillation, the CHADS2 score (Table 13.2) is a validated clinical prediction score that uses congestive heart failure, hypertension, age >75 years, diabetes and history of

TABLE 13.1
Oral Anticoagulants and Antiplatelet Agents

Drugs	Mechanism of Action	Dosage	Stopping Medication Before Surgery
Warfarin	Vitamin K antagonist	Widely varies	Withheld for approximately 5 days
Dabigatran (Pradaxa)	Direct thrombin inhibitors	150 mg BD for most patients; 110 mg BD for age >75, CrCl 30–49 mL/min	Between 24 h in low-bleeding-risk patients with a normal renal function to >96 h in a high-risk individual with impaired renal function
Rivaroxaban (Xarelto)	Factor Xa inhibitor	20 mg daily for most patients; 15 mg daily if CrCl 30–49 mL/min; avoid if CrCl <30 mL/min	24–48 h
Apixaban (Eliquis)	Factor Xa inhibitor	5 mg BD for most patients; for age >80 years, weight <60 kg, S creat >133 µL/L may require 2.5 mg BD	24–48 h
Aspirin	Inhibits thromboxane A_2 synthesis by irreversibly acetylating cyclooxygenase-1 in platelets and megakaryocyte	75–325 mg once daily	Most often can be continued; may need to be stopped 7 days before surgery
Clopidogrel	Clopidogrel is metabolised in the liver to active compounds which covalently bind to the ADP receptors on platelets and reduce platelet activation	75 mg daily	7 days prior to surgery
Prasugrel	An ADP receptor antagonist	Adults >60 kg: 10 mg once daily; <60 kg: 5 mg once daily	7 days prior to surgery
Ticagrelor	Reversible, direct-acting inhibitor of the adenosine diphosphate receptor P2Y12	90 mg twice daily	5 days prior to surgery

Some variation exists in the recommended time to cease dabigatran between the European Society of Cardiology guidelines and the Queensland Health guidelines. The latter guidelines recommend stopping dabigatran for 5 days in patients with CrCl of 31–50 mL/min, and greater than 5 days (and not to restart) in patients with CrCl <30 mL/min
ADP=adenosine diphosphate; CrCl=creatinine clearance.; S creat=serum creatinine.
(Reproduced with permission from Rahman A, Latona J. New oral anticoagulants and perioperative management of anticoagulant/antiplatelet agents. *Aust Fam Physician* 2014;43(12):2014.)

stroke or transient ischaemic attack in a cumulative manner to estimate expected stroke rate per 100-patient years.[3] Thus, patients with high CHADS2 scores would be considered at high risk of thrombosis. (See also Table 12.4.)

- Early data suggest that the CHADS2 score may also be used to predict risk for postsurgical stroke. Kaatz and colleagues[4] showed, in a population-based, retrospective cohort study involving 37,469 patients

with AF, that 401 (1.1%) developed a stroke within 30 days of non-cardiac surgery compared with 7260 (0.3%) in 2,228,360 patients without AF ($P<0.001$). The 30-day risk for postoperative stroke increased with each point score in the CHADS2 score.[4]

- Patients with mechanical heart valves are also at increased risk of systemic embolisation and occlusive thrombus of the orifice of the prosthetic valve during subtherapeutic levels of warfarin.[5] Older, caged-ball

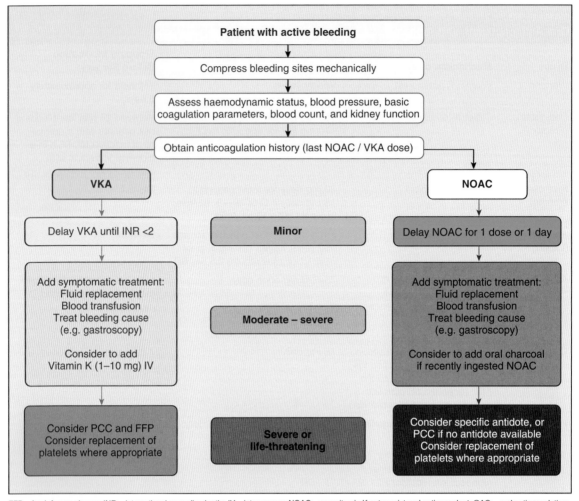

FFP = fresh frozen plasma; INR = international normalized ratio; IV = intravenous; NOAC = non-vitamin K antagonist oral anticoagulant; OAC = oral anticoagulation; PCC = prothrombin complex concentrates; VKA = vitamin K antagonist.

FIG. 13.1 Management of active bleeding in patients receiving anticoagulation. Institutions should have an agreed procedure in place. (Reproduced with permission from Kirchhof P, Benussi S, Kotecha D, Ahlsson A, Atar D, Casadei B, et al.; ESC Scientific Document Group. 2016 ESC Guidelines for the management of atrial fibrillation developed in collaboration with EACTS. Eur Heart J 2016;37(38):2925, Fig 11.)

valves are the most thrombogenic, followed by tilting-disc valves. Bileaflet valves are the least thrombogenic.[6] The risk of thromboembolic events is greatest in the first 3 months after implantation.

- The intensity of antithrombotic therapy in patients with a mechanical prosthesis is guided by the type of prosthesis, its position and other patient-related risk factors (Table 13.3).[7]
- Thromboembolic events are more common with prosthetic mitral valves than with aortic valves. In the absence of anticoagulant therapy, mitral position

valves have an annualised risk of thrombosis of 22% compared with aortic position valves, with an annualised risk of approximately 10%–12%.[8]

- The anticoagulation strategy selected depends upon an evaluation of the thromboembolic risk and the haemorrhagic risk of the surgical procedure.

The American College of Chest Physicians' *Antithrombotic therapy and prevention of thrombosis* evidence-based clinical practice guidelines suggest a clinically useful thromboembolic risk stratification in the periprocedural period, as shown in Table 13.4.[8]

TABLE 13.2
CHADS2 Score and Adjusted Risk of Stroke

CHADS2 SCORE

C	Congestive heart failure	1 point
H	Hypertension	1 point
A	Age >75 years	1 point
D	Diabetes	1 point
S2	Stroke	2 points

ADJUSTED RISK OF STROKE FOR CHADS2 SCORE

Score	Adjusted Risk of Stroke per Year (%)
0	1.9
1	2.8
2	4
3	5.9
4	8.5
5	12.5
6	18.2

Low-bleeding-risk procedures

- VKAs may be continued in those with relatively low INR 1.5–1.8 for minor procedures with a low risk of bleeding.[9]
- These include excision of skin lesions, cataract surgery and procedures in which the bleeding can be controlled readily by local measures. This approach is not recommended for laparoscopic surgery, ultrasound or CT-guided biopsies.

High-bleeding-risk procedures

- The strategy for perioperative anticoagulation in patients undergoing major, high-bleeding-risk surgery is based on the assessment of the risk of thromboembolism versus the risk of haemorrhage.
- In the low-thromboembolism-risk group, warfarin can be withheld for 5 days before surgery without any bridging anticoagulation with unfractionated or low-molecular-weight heparin.
- Generally, high-thromboembolism-risk patients should be considered for more-aggressive perioperative management strategy with bridging therapy. With regards to warfarin, a relatively normal zone of haemostasis exists when the INR is 1.0–2.0.[10]

TABLE 13.3
Prosthetic Heart Valves: Need and Intensity for the Anticoagulation Therapy[7]

Valve Type	Cardiac Impairment	Target INR
Bioprosthetic (mitral or aortic)	No	2.5 (range 2.0–3.0) for first 3 months following valve replacement followed by long-term aspirin daily
	Atrial fibrillation	2.5 (range 2.0–3.0) indefinitely
	History of systemic embolism	2.5 (range 2.0–3.0) for 3–12 months
	Left atrial thrombus at time of surgery	2.5 (range 2.0–3.0) long-term but duration uncertain
MECHANICAL		
Aortic mechanical bileaflet valves	No	2.5 (range 2.0–3.0) indefinitely
Aortic mechanical bileaflet valves	Atrial fibrillation	3.0 (range 2.0–3.5) indefinitely or 2.5 (range 2.0–3.0) plus low-dose aspirin
Mechanical bileaflet and tilting-disc mitral valves		3.0 (range 2.5–3.5) indefinitely or 2.5 (range 2.0–3.0) plus low-dose aspirin
Caged-ball or caged-disc valves		3.0 (range 2.5–3.5) indefinitely
Mechanical valve	Additional risk factors including previous systemic embolism whilst on warfarin	3.0 (range 2.5–3.5) indefinitely plus low-dose aspirin

AF = atrial fibrillation.

TABLE 13.4
Risk of Thromboembolism in Patients on Warfarin

Risk Stratum	Indication of Warfarin Therapy		
	Mechanical Heart Valve	*Atrial Fibrillation*	*Venous Thromboembolism (VTE)*
High	• Any mitral valve prosthesis • Any caged-ball or tilting-disc aortic valve prosthesis • Recent (within 6 months) stroke or transient ischaemic attack	• CHADS2 score of 5 or 6 • Recent (within 3 months) stroke or transient ischaemic attack • Rheumatic valvular heart disease	• Recent (within 3 months) VTE • Severe thrombophilia (e.g. deficiency of protein C, protein S or antithrombin; antiphospholipid antibodies; multiple abnormalities)
Moderate	• Bileaflet aortic valve prosthesis and one or more of the following risk factors: atrial fibrillation, prior stroke or transient ischaemic attack, hypertension, diabetes, congestive heart failure, age >75 years	• CHADS2 score of 3 or 4	• VTE within the past 3–12 months • Non-severe thrombophilia (e.g. heterozygous factor V Leiden or prothrombin gene mutation) • Recurrent VTE • Active cancer (treated within 6 months or palliative)
Low	• Bileaflet aortic valve prosthesis without atrial fibrillation and no other risk factors for stroke	• CHADS2 score of 0–2 (assuming no prior stroke or transient ischaemic attack)	• VTE >12 months previous and no other risk factors

(Reproduced with permission from Latona J, Rahman A. Management of oral anticoagulation in the surgical patient. *ANZ J Surg* 2015;85:620–5.)

• Although the INR value at which the risk of bleeding increases is not known, the risk is assumed not to be elevated when the INR <1.5, and elevated when the INR is more than 2.0.[8]
• When bridging therapy is needed for patients at high risk, unfractionated heparin is preferred when the creatinine clearance (CrCl) is less than 30. In procedures when bridging therapy is required, the usual protocol is to stop warfarin 5 days before the procedure and to start low-molecular-weight heparin at a therapeutic dose once the INR <2.[11]
• The INR is usually checked on the morning of the procedure, whereas enoxaparin should be last given 24 hours prior to the procedure. Unfractionated heparin, on the other hand, is usually stopped 4–6 hours before high-risk procedures.[8]

Non-vitamin K antagonist oral anticoagulants During Surgery
• Patient factors, such as renal function, age, history of bleeding complications, concomitant medications and surgical factors, should be taken into account prior to discontinuing the drug. Compared with warfarin, which may need bridging anticoagulation in patients with higher thromboembolic risks (see Table 13.2), patients on NOACs are less likely to require bridging therapy.[12] This is explained by the short half-life, which allows for properly timed short-term cessation and early re-initiation after surgery.
• In the case of emergency, surgery should ideally be deferred for 12–24 hours (since the last dose) if possible. If not, then a multidisciplinary team approach including a surgeon, haematologist and cardiologist should be considered, and the risk of bleeding carefully assessed and discussed with the patient and relatives. These should be assessed on a case-by-case basis.
• Most of these novel drugs do not have specific antidotes and management of bleeding is thus largely supportive. It should be remembered that, unlike warfarin (where the activity of the drug can be monitored by INR), there are currently limited lab

tests that can predict the risk of bleeding while on a NOAC. The activated partial thromboplastin time (aPTT) provides a qualitative assessment of the presence of a direct thrombin inhibitor (dabigatran). Similarly, the prothrombin time (PT) may provide a qualitative assessment of the presence of factor Xa inhibitors (rivaroxaban, apixaban). Unfortunately, neither of these tests is sensitive for quantitative assessment of NOAC effect.

Anticoagulation reversal during urgent surgery

- Urgent warfarin reversal requires replacement of the clotting factors. Prothrombin complex concentrate reverses warfarin within 15 minutes. Fresh frozen plasma also has a rapid onset of action but duration of action is short. Vitamin K given intravenously has an onset of action in 6–8 hours but has sustained action.
- Idarucizumab is a humanised monoclonal antibody that binds to both free and thrombin-bound dabigatran and fully reverses its anticoagulation effects. It does not have any inherent prothrombotic effects. Idarucizumab does not reverse either rivaroxaban or apixaban.[13]
- Besides idarucizumab, other reversal agents are in development for the reversal of both dabigatran and the other NOACs. These include andexanet alfa, a recombinant truncated form of enzymatically inactive factor Xa, which binds and reverses the anticoagulant action of the factor Xa inhibitors.[14]

Restarting Non-vitamin K antagonist oral anticoagulants After Surgery

- The timing to restart the NOACS after surgery will depend on multiple factors. These include the factors mentioned above, along with the type of surgery and the ability to achieve immediate haemostasis. Again, the risk of bleeding should be weighed against the risk of thromboembolism. For procedures with immediate and complete haemostasis, NOACs can be resumed 6–8 hours after intervention.
- In many surgical interventions, the resumption of anticoagulation within 48–72 hours may carry significant bleeding risk and therefore is better off deferred. Once NOACs are restarted, maximal anticoagulation will be obtained within 2 hours.

Non-vitamin-K Antagonist Oral Anticoagulants vs Warfarin

- The NOACs so far tested in clinical trials have all shown non-inferiority compared with VKAs, and

with better safety, consistently reducing the number of intracranial haemorrhages.[15] On this basis, the 2012 focused update of the ESC guidelines for the management of atrial fibrillation now recommend them as 'broadly preferable to VKA in the vast majority of patients with non-valvular atrial fibrillation' (see Box 13.1).

- Generally, stable patients taking warfarin whose INRs are largely within the targeted therapeutic range, and in whom INR testing does not present a problem, may prefer to continue with warfarin. If a particular patient does have difficulties maintaining INR results within the therapeutic range, switching to a new oral anticoagulant is an option to consider and the postoperative setting may be the perfect opportunity to address the issue.

Factors to Consider Before Switching From Warfarin to NOAC After Surgery

1. Renal function

Before switching from warfarin to NOAC, one of the most important considerations should be one's renal function. In the presence of significant renal impairment (estimated glomerular filtration rate <30 mL/min) most of the NOACs are contraindicated. In the presence of a moderate renal impairment, NOAC should be used with caution and, in most cases, dosages need to be reduced.

2. Compliance

Compliance and adherence to treatment are crucial, especially as these drugs have a relatively short half-life.

3. INR

When switching from a VKA to a NOAC, the INR should be allowed to fall to less than 2.0 before starting the NOAC.

PERIOPERATIVE MANAGEMENT OF ANTIPLATELET THERAPY

- Dual antiplatelet therapy following percutaneous coronary stenting and acute coronary syndrome is common. Antiplatelet medications that are used commonly in Australia include aspirin, clopidogrel, prasugrel and ticagrelor (see Table 13.1). Management of patients on DAPT who are referred for surgical procedures depends on the level of emergency and the thrombotic and bleeding risk of the individual patient. Antiplatelet therapy interruption may expose patients to the potential risk of stent thrombosis, perioperative myocardial infarction or cardiovascular death, whereas continuing these agents is often associated with increased bleeding.

- The current recommendation for DAPT (with aspirin and clopidogrel) is for 6 months in patients undergoing elective stenting (for chronic coronary syndrome), irrespective of stent type, unless a shorter duration (1–3 months) is indicated because of the risk or occurrence of life-threatening bleeding. In this situation, clopidogrel 75 mg daily should be considered for 3 months in patients with a higher risk of life-threatening bleeding, and for 1 month in patients with very high risk of life-threatening bleeding.[16]

- DAPT in the form of aspirin and a P2Y12 inhibitor (ticagrelor, prasugrel or clopidogrel) is recommended for 12 months after percutaneous coronary intervention (PCI) following ACS, unless there are contraindications. In patients who are at high risk of bleeding, discontinuation of P2Y12 inhibitor therapy after 6 months should be considered.[17]

- In some cases of complex stenting (e.g. bifurcation stenting) continuation of DAPT for longer than 1 year may be necessary. Premature cessation of DAPT is thought to be one of the most important causes of stent thrombosis, which can have fatal consequences.[18]

- Patients requiring surgery within 12 months after drug-eluting stent PCI (DES-PCI) had an increased risk of myocardial infarction and cardiac death. The increased risk is mostly present within the first month after DES-PCI, suggesting that surgery might be undertaken earlier than is currently recommended.[19]

- For patients at high thrombotic and high haemorrhagic risk, postponement of elective surgery should be considered. If surgery cannot be deferred, aspirin should be continued while discontinuing P2Y12 receptor inhibitor. P2Y12 could be reintroduced with a loading dose within 24–72 hours after haemostasis is achieved. Bridging with a short-acting intravenous antiplatelet therapy (a2b3a inhibitor) could be considered.

- Perioperative continuation of aspirin increases bleeding risk slightly, but does not increase the risk for bleeding that required medical or other interventions, and therefore can usually be continued.[20,21] On the other hand, perioperative interruption of aspirin confers a threefold increased risk for adverse cardiovascular events.[22]

- Proposed bridging protocols for patients on dual antiplatelet therapy with aspirin plus a P2Y12 receptor inhibitor referred to cardiac or non-cardiac surgery are given in Fig. 13.2.[23]

If a patient is to undergo high-bleeding-risk surgery and an antiplatelet effect is not desired, clopidogrel, prasugrel and ticagrelor should be discontinued 5–7 days prior to the procedure.[16,24]

Good communication with the treating cardiologist and, in some cases, an individualised treatment plan may be necessary for managing such patients in the perioperative period.

CONCLUSION

- The strategy of management of anticoagulation/antiplatelet agents in the perioperative period is based on the assessment of each patient's thromboembolic and bleeding risks. Most patients having minor procedures can continue to take anticoagulants, provided that they are closely monitored. High-thrombotic-risk patients should be considered for more aggressive perioperative management strategy with bridging therapy.

- Antiplatelet therapy is usually safe to continue in low-bleeding-risk procedures. Generally, drugs like clopidogrel, prasugrel and ticagrelor should be stopped around 5–7 days prior to any procedure where the risk of bleeding is deemed to be high. Low-dose aspirin alone does not substantially increase the risk of clinically important bleeding after invasive procedures and can usually be continued during surgery.

- The timing of any non-urgent procedure and stopping of antiplatelet therapy depends on the time frame between the insertion of stents and the planned procedure, and on whether or not the stent was inserted following acute coronary syndrome.

Based on the above, Mr Johnson does not necessarily need to discontinue his NOAC as the risk of bleeding is small. If there were concerns about increased risk of bleeding, then the best approach would be to stop the rivaroxaban 24 hours prior to the procedure and take the next dose the morning after the procedure.

Mr Smith should not have cessation of his DAPT. His angioplasty was performed only 2 weeks prior and, as the risk of bleeding is low, DAPT should be continued. If the risk of bleeding in the procedure were deemed to be high on DAPT, then the procedure would be better off postponed until a time when it is deemed safe to stop his clopidogrel.

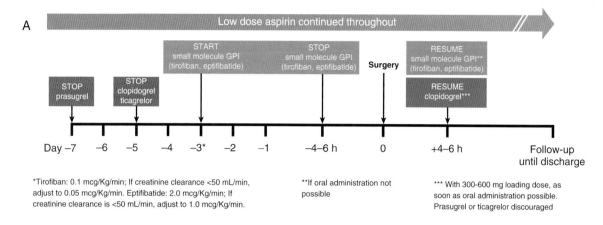

*Tirofiban: 0.1 mcg/Kg/min; If creatinine clearance <50 mL/min, adjust to 0.05 mcg/Kg/min. Eptifibatide: 2.0 mcg/Kg/min; If creatinine clearance is <50 mL/min, adjust to 1.0 mcg/Kg/min.

**If oral administration not possible

*** With 300-600 mg loading dose, as soon as oral administration possible. Prasugrel or ticagrelor discouraged

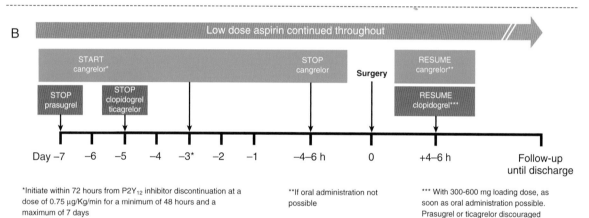

*Initiate within 72 hours from P2Y$_{12}$ inhibitor discontinuation at a dose of 0.75 µg/Kg/min for a minimum of 48 hours and a maximum of 7 days

**If oral administration not possible

*** With 300-600 mg loading dose, as soon as oral administration possible. Prasugrel or ticagrelor discouraged

FIG. 13.2 Proposed bridging protocols for patients on dual antiplatelet therapy with aspirin plus a P2Y12 receptor inhibitor referred to cardiac or non-cardiac surgery. **(A)** Bridging strategy with small-molecule glycoprotein IIb/IIIa inhibitors (GPI). **(B)** Bridging strategy with cangrelor. (Reproduced with permission from Capodanno D, Angiolillo DJ. Management of antiplatelet therapy in patients with coronary artery disease requiring cardiac and noncardiac surgery. Circulation 2013;128:2785–98.)

REFERENCES

1. Pharmaceutical Benefits Scheme. http://www.pbs.gov.au/pbs/search?term=noacs&search-type=info.
2. Healey JS, Eikelboom J, Douketis J, Wallentin L, Oldgren J, Yang S, et al. Periprocedural bleeding and thromboembolic events with dabigatran compared to warfarin: results from the RE-LY Randomized Trial. Circulation 2012;126:343–8.
3. Gage BF, Waterman AD, Shannon W, Boechler M, Rich MW, Radford MJ. Validation of clinical classification schemes for predicting stroke: results from the National Registry of Atrial Fibrillation. JAMA 2001;285:2864–70.
4. Kaatz S, Douketis JD, White RH, Zhou H. Can the CHADS2 score predict postoperative stroke risk in patients with chronic atrial fibrillation who are having elective non-cardiac surgery? J Thromb Haemost 2011;9:P-WE-367.
5. Cannegieter SC, Rosendaal FR, Briet E. Thromboembolic and bleeding complications in patients with mechanical heart valve prostheses. Circulation 1994;89(2):635–41.
6. Ansell J, Hirsh J, Poller L, Bussey H, Jacobson A, Hylek E. The pharmacology and management of the vitamin K antagonists: the Seventh ACCP Conference on antithrombotic and thrombolytic therapy. Chest 2004;126(3 Suppl.):204S–33S.
7. Stein PD, Alpert JS, Dalen JE, Horstkotte D, Turpie AG. Antithrombotic therapy in patients with mechanical and biological prosthetic heart valves. Chest 1998;114:602S–10S.
8. Douketis JD, Spyropoulos AC, Spencer FA, Mayr M, Jaffer AK, Eckman MH, et al. Perioperative management of antithrombotic therapy: Antithrombotic therapy and prevention of thrombosis, 9th ed: American College of Chest Physicians Evidence-based clinical practice guidelines. Chest 2012;141(2 Suppl.):e326S–50S.

9. Rustad H, Myhre E. Surgery during anticoagulant treatment. The risk of increased bleeding in patients on oral anticoagulant treatment. *Acta Med Scand* 1963;**173**:115–19.

10. Dzik WS. Reversal of drug-induced anticoagulation: old solutions and new problems. *Transfusion* 2012;**52**(Suppl. 1):45S–55S.

11. Baron TH, Kamath PS, McBane RD. Management of antithrombotic therapy in patients undergoing invasive procedures. *N Engl J Med* 2013;**368**:22.

12. Heidbuchel H, Verhamme P, Alings M, Antz M, Hacke W, Oldgren J, et al; European Heart Rhythm Association. European Heart Rhythm Association practical guide on the use of new oral anticoagulants in patients with non-valvular AF. *Europace* 2013;**15**:625–51.

13. Eikelboom JW, Quinlan DJ, van Ryn J, Weitz JI. Idarucizumab – the antidote for reversal of dabigatran. *Circulation* 2015;**132**:2412–22.

14. Greinacher A, Thiele T, Selleng K. Reversal of anticoagulants: an overview of current developments. *Thromb Haemost* 2015;**113**:931–42.

15. Ruff CT, Giugliano RP, Braunwald E, Hoffman EB, Deenadayalu N, Ezekowitz MD, et al. Comparison of the efficacy and safety of new oral anticoagulants with warfarin in patients with atrial fibrillation: a meta-analysis of randomised trials. *Lancet* 2014;**383**(9921):955–62.

16. Valgimigli M, Bueno H, Byrne RA, Collet JP, Costa F, Jeppsson A, et al; ESC Scientific Document Group; ESC Committee for Practice Guidelines (CPG); ESC National Cardiac Societies. 2017 ESC focused update on dual anti-platelet therapy in coronary artery disease developed in collaboration with EACTS: the Task Force for dual antiplatelet therapy in coronary artery disease of the European Society of Cardiology (ESC) and of the European Association for Cardio-Thoracic Surgery (EACTS). *Eur Heart J* 2018;**39**:213–60.

17. Chew DP, Scott IA, Cullen L, French JK, Briffa TG, Tideman PA, et al; NHFA/CSANZ ACS Guideline 2016 Executive Working Group. National Heart Foundation of Australia & Cardiac Society of Australia and New Zealand: Australian clinical guidelines for the management of acute coronary syndromes 2016. *Heart Lung Circ* 2016;**25**:895–951.

18. Iakovou I, Schmidt T, Bonizzoni E, Ge L, Sangiorgi GM, Stankovic G, et al. Incidence, predictors, and outcome of thrombosis after successful implantation of drug-eluting stents. *JAMA* 2005;**293**:2126–30.

19. Egholm G, Kristensen SD, Thim T, Olesen KK, Madsen M, Jensen SE, et al. Risk associated with surgery within 12 months after coronary drug-eluting stent implantation. *J Am Coll Cardiol* 2016;**68**:2622–32.

20. Burger W, Chemnitius JM, Kneissl GD. Rücker G. Low-dose aspirin for secondary cardiovascular prevention – cardiovascular risks after its perioperative withdrawal versus bleeding risks with its continuation – review and meta-analysis. *J Intern Med* 2005;**257**(5):399.

21. Carmignani L, Picozzi S, Bozzini G, Negri E, Ricci C, Gaeta M, et al. Transrectal ultrasound-guided prostate biopsies in patients taking aspirin for cardiovascular disease: a meta-analysis. *Transfus Apher Sci* 2011;**45**:275–80.

22. Biondi-Zoccai GG, Lotrionte M, Agostoni P, Abbate A, Fusaro M, Burzotta F, et al. A systematic review and meta-analysis on the hazards of discontinuing or not adhering to aspirin among 50,279 patients at risk for coronary artery disease. *Eur Heart J* 2006;**27**(22):2667–74.

23. Capodanno D, Angiolillo DJ. Management of anti-platelet therapy in patients with coronary artery disease requiring cardiac and noncardiac surgery. *Circulation* 2013;**128**:2785–98.

24. Wallentin L, Becker RC, Budaj A, Cannon CP, Emanuelsson H, Held C, et al; PLATO Investigators, Freij A, Thorsén M. Ticagrelor versus clopidogrel in patients with acute coronary syndromes. *N Engl J Med* 2009;**361**:1045–57.

CHAPTER 14

Hypertension

KEY POINTS

- Hypertension is a major modifiable risk factor for cardiovascular diseases and stroke, and an important cause of premature death.
- The diagnosis of hypertension should be based on multiple office blood pressure (BP) measurements taken on at least on two separate occasions.
- The assessment of someone with hypertension should include a detailed medical history, physical examination and assessment of absolute cardiovascular risk.
- The cause of primary hypertension is not clearly known, although genetic and environmental factors may play a significant role.
- Primary hyperaldosteronism is the most common cause of secondary hypertension.
- Lifestyle interventions, including increased physical activity and a healthy balanced diet with reduced salt intake, are important for successful BP control.
- In addition to lifestyle changes, the majority of patients require pharmacotherapy to achieve optimum BP control.
- The choice of drugs should be influenced by the age, ethnicity, race and other clinical characteristics, including co-existing medical conditions of the patient.
- The majority of patients require a combination therapy to achieve contemporary BP targets.
- The aim should be to target BP to 130/80 mmHg for most patients, if tolerated.

CASE 17 SCENARIO: DAVID WITH LEFT VENTRICULAR HYPERTROPHY

63-year-old David has come to the surgery for review. Two weeks previously he was reviewed for an upper respiratory tract infection and was found to have a BP of 148/93 mmHg. He is a smoker and has history of type II diabetes which is well controlled on metformin 1 g daily.

Today his BP is 149/96 mmHg. His ECG shows sinus rhythm with left ventricular hypertrophy on voltage criteria. His physical examination is otherwise unremarkable. His dipstick urine test did not show any glycosuria or proteinuria.

David was prescribed perindopril 5 mg daily at bedtime and advised on a healthy active lifestyle. He was also advised to adopt a diet low in sodium and saturated fat, and to increase his intake of fruits and vegetables. He had routine blood tests, including renal function tests, electrolytes, fasting lipid profile and glucose, and had a chest x-ray arranged.

Hypertension is one of the most important preventable causes of premature death worldwide. In 2014/15, 34% of Australians aged 18 years and over had high BP or were taking antihypertensive medications.[1]

There is a close relationship between blood pressure and the risk of cardiovascular events, strokes and mortality. Cardiovascular mortality doubles with each 20/10 mmHg increase in BP.[2] In a meta-analysis involving 123 studies with 613,815 patients, overall a 10 mmHg reduction of systolic BP reduced the risk of major cardiovascular disease events by 20%, coronary heart disease by 17%, heart failure by 28% and all-cause mortality by 13%.[3]

DEFINITION OF HYPERTENSION

- Most major guidelines recommend that hypertension be diagnosed when a person's systolic BP is ≥140 mmHg or the diastolic BP is ≥90 mmHg, or both, on repeated examination.
- The 2016 National Heart Foundation of Australia guidelines for the diagnosis and management of hypertension in adults[4] and the 2018 ESC/ESH practice guidelines for the management of arterial hypertension[5] maintain traditional BP categories, with grade 1 hypertension starting at an office pressure of 140/90 mmHg (Table 14.1). However,

TABLE 14.1
Classification of Clinic Blood Pressure Levels in Adults[4]

Diagnostic Category	Systolic Blood Pressure (mmHg)
Grade 1 hypertension	140–59
Grade 2 hypertension	160–79
Grade 3 hypertension	>180

the 2017 ACC/AHA guidelines for the prevention, detection, evaluation and management of high BP in adults[6] have lowered the threshold for stage 1 hypertension to 130/80 mmHg and recommend lowering BP to less than 130/80 mmHg for all adults.

- The 2018 ESC/ESH practice guidelines for the management of arterial hypertension in adults define hypertension as a persistent elevation in office systolic BP ≥140 and/or diastolic BP ≥90 mmHg, which is equivalent to a 24-hour ambulatory blood pressure monitoring (ABPM) average of ≥130/80 mmHg or a home BP monitoring average ≥135/85 mmHg.[5]

The assessment of someone with hypertension should include a detailed medical history, physical examination, assessment of absolute cardiovascular risk, basic laboratory investigations and further diagnostic tests when appropriate. The aim of the diagnostic process is to:
- identify overall cardiovascular risk factors and co-morbidities
- detect end-organ damage
- investigate for causes of secondary hypertension when appropriate.

HYPERTENSIVE EMERGENCIES

These include:
- malignant hypertension – grade 3 hypertension, associated with fundoscopic changes including haemorrhage, exudates with or without papilloedema and, at times, heart failure, encephalopathy or acute kidney injury
- hypertension-associated acute aortic dissection or acute myocardial infarction
- patients with severe hypertension due to phaeochromocytoma
- pregnancy-induced severe hypertension or pre-eclampsia.

CONFIRMING THE DIAGNOSIS OF HYPERTENSION

- The diagnosis of hypertension should be based on multiple office BP measurements taken on at least two separate occasions, preferably on both arms using an appropriately sized cuff, or by out-of-office measurement using ABPM, or by home BP monitoring.
- Clinic BP measurement can be affected by stress. White coat hypertension refers to the finding of elevated clinic BP but normal readings on ABPM or by self-monitoring of BP outside the office setting.
- ABPM usually measures BP every 30 minutes over a 24-hour period while patients continue normal daily activities, including (if possible) sleep. ABPM provides the average daytime and night-time BP readings. These are a better predictor of cardiovascular outcomes than clinic BP. The night-time average BP should be at least 10% lower than the daytime average (dippers). Absence of nocturnal BP dipping (non-dippers) can be seen in sleep apnoea, older age and autonomic dysfunction.
- ABPM values are, generally, lower than those of clinic BP values and the diagnostic threshold for hypertension is >130/80 mmHg.

PRIMARY AND SECONDARY HYPERTENSION

Primary (Idiopathic or Essential[1]) Hypertension

- This was called *essential* because it was thought elevated BP was necessary for adequate perfusion of atherosclerotic arteries.
- The cause of primary hypertension is not clearly known, although genetic and environmental factors may play a significant role. Environmental factors including poor diet, excess intake of salt, insufficient intake of potassium, obesity, sedentary lifestyle, and excessive alcohol consumption are all contributors to hypertension. About 95% of adults with high BP have primary hypertension.

Secondary Hypertension

- Secondary hypertension is elevated BP that results from an underlying, identifiable cause. This pertains to the relatively small number of cases, about 5% of all hypertension, where the cause of the high BP can be identified and sometimes treated.[7]
- The main causes of secondary hypertension are renal parenchymal disease, renovascular disease, primary aldosteronism, obstructive sleep apnoea, drug and

TABLE 14.2
Findings That Suggest Secondary Hypertension

Primary hyperaldosteronism is the most common cause of secondary hypertension. The patient may have spontaneous or diuretic-induced hypokalaemia, incidental findings of an adrenal mass and high aldosterone/renin ratio (screening test).	Primary aldosteronism
There may be a history of snoring, daytime somnolence and obesity. A 24-hour ambulatory BP may show loss of nocturnal dipping.	Sleep apnoea
The serum creatinine may be elevated with or without proteinuria and haematuria. An enlarged kidney may be palpated in a patient with polycystic kidney disease.	Renal parenchymal disease
Fibromuscular dysplasia should be suspected in a young female with hypertension. There may be a renal bruit. Atherosclerotic renal artery stenosis is common in the older patients who are vasculopaths, present with increasing difficult to control BP and episodes of flash pulmonary oedema. Renal artery duplex ultrasound and CT renal angiography are diagnostic.	Renovascular disease
These patients may present with paroxysmal hypertension superimposed on sustained hypertension, diaphoresis, headache and palpitations. Elevated plasma metanephrines or elevated 24-hour urinary catecholamines are keys to diagnosing phaeochromocytoma.	Phaeochromocytoma
There may be a history of use of oral contraceptives, excessive alcohol, caffeine, non-steroidal anti-inflammatory drugs, corticosteroids or cyclosporine, certain antidepressants (e.g. MAO inhibitors) or an atypical antipsychotic (e.g. clozapine). Illicit drugs including cocaine and amphetamines can be a cause. Certain herbal agents also can cause hypertension.	Drug or alcohol induced
These patients may present with a higher BP in upper extremities than in lower extremities. There may be radiofemoral delay, a murmur and an abnormal chest x-ray. An echocardiogram or CT aortogram may be diagnostic.	Coarctation of aorta

BP=blood pressure; MAO=mono amine oxidase.

alcohol consumption, renal artery stenosis and phaeochromocytoma.
- Screening for secondary hypertension should be considered when the onset of hypertension is at <30 years of age, when the clinical features listed in Table 14.2 are present and in adults with resistant hypertension.

PHYSICAL EXAMINATION

- Blood pressure should be measured using an appropriately sized cuff, when the patient is fully relaxed and preferably in both arms.
- Body mass index and waist circumference should be measured.
- Fundoscopy is indicated to look for retinal haemorrhages, papilloedema and other signs of hypertensive retinopathy.
- A complete cardiovascular examination should include assessment of:
  - *pulse:*
    - rate, rhythm, volume, character, radiofemoral delay

  - auscultation of the carotid and femoral arteries, for the presence of a bruit
  - *signs of heart failure:*
    - jugular venous pressure, an added heart sound
    - crackles on pulmonary auscultation
    - peripheral oedema
  - *examination of the abdomen for:*
    - polycystic kidneys, renal bruits
  - *signs of:*
    - Cushing's syndrome, thyroid disease
  - *dipstick urine for:*
    - proteinuria, haematuria.

CLINICAL INVESTIGATIONS

- A standard 12-lead ECG is indicated to screen for left ventricular hypertrophy (Fig. 14.1) and to document heart rate and rhythm.
- An echocardiogram is recommended to evaluate cardiac structure and function because this might influence treatment, including the choice of antihypertensive medications. Echocardiography is particularly important when there is evidence of left ventricular

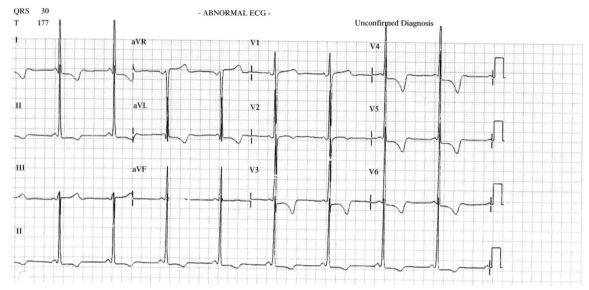

FIG. 14.1 ECG in a patient with left ventricular hypertrophy showing high amplitude of the QRS segment, ST-segment depression and asymmetrical T-wave inversion.

hypertrophy or intraventricular conduction abnormality on the ECG.

- Chronic kidney disease is an important cause of secondary hypertension and, hence, serum creatinine measurement is recommended. The patient should also have haemoglobin, fasting blood glucose, HbA_{1c}, fasting lipid profile, electrolytes and liver function tests, urine analysis and the urine albumin: creatinine ratio assessed.
- Ultrasound examination of the carotid arteries can be considered to exclude asymptomatic atherosclerosis, particularly in older patients.
- Ankle–brachial index (ABI) is indicated especially in those with clinical suspicion of peripheral vascular disease. An ABI <0.9 is diagnostic of peripheral vascular disease.

MANAGEMENT

Non-Pharmacological

Lifestyle interventions are important because they can complement the blood pressure-lowering effect of drug treatment and delay the need for drug treatment initiation.[5]

Exercise and blood pressure

- Increased physical activity by means of a structured exercise program is recommended for adults with elevated BP. A systematic review of randomised controlled trials of lifestyle interventions to reduce raised BP showed statistically significant benefits for aerobic exercise, with mean reductions in systolic BP of 4.6 mmHg and corresponding reductions in diastolic BP.[8]
- A systematic review and meta-analysis, involving 15 randomised controlled trials of the beneficial effects of endurance exercise on ambulatory BP, suggestsed that aerobic endurance exercise significantly decreases (systolic BP 3.2 mmHg, diastolic BP 2.7 mmHg) during daytime, but not night-time, ambulatory BP measurement.[9]
- The hypertensive patient should be advised to participate in at least 30 minutes of moderate-intensity dynamic exercise (walking, jogging, cycling or swimming) for 5–7 days a week.[5]

Diet

- Hypertensive patients (and indeed all patients) should be advised to eat a healthy balanced diet containing vegetables, fresh fruits, low-fat dairy products, fish and unsaturated fatty acids.
- The established dietary modifications that are proven to lower blood pressure are contained in the DASH (Dietary Approaches to Stop Hypertension) diet, recommended for adults with hypertension.[10]
- In the randomised controlled PREDIMED trial, a Mediterranean diet supplemented with extra virgin olive oil or nuts reduced 24-hour ambulatory BP,

total cholesterol and fasting glucose in high-risk individuals.[11]

Salt intake

- There is evidence of a causal relationship between sodium intake and blood pressure. Sodium restriction has been shown to lower both systolic and diastolic BP, particularly in hypertensive patients.
- A Cochrane review of 167 studies assessing the effect of low sodium intake on BP reduction found a 1% decrease in BP in normotensives and a 3.5% decrease in hypertensive patients. Effects on BP reduction were more pronounced in Asian populations than in Caucasians.[12]
- The 2016 Australian guidelines[4] recommend reduction of salt intake to <6 g/day for primary prevention (i.e. for normotensive patients) and <4 g/day for secondary prevention.
- Unless the patient has a contraindication due to chronic kidney disease, or is taking a medication that can precipitate hyperkalaemia, potassium supplementation, preferably via dietary modification, is recommended for adults with elevated BP.
- Dietary potassium intake is inversely related to BP. Increasing dietary potassium can reduce systolic BP by 4–8 mmHg in patients with hypertension and about 2 mmHg in normotensive subjects.[13]

Alcohol consumption

- The risk for hypertension increases linearly with alcohol consumption in both men and women. Consumption of more than two standard drinks a day for men and more than one standard drink for women has been found to be associated with an increased risk of developing hypertension.[14]
- Adult men and women with elevated BP or hypertension who currently consume alcohol should be advised to drink no more than two and one standard drinks per day, respectively.[6]

Weight reduction

- Increased body weight is an important risk factor for hypertension. Weight loss is recommended to reduce BP in adults with hypertension who are overweight.
- A meta-analysis of randomised controlled trials performed to estimate the effect of weight reduction on BP control has shown that a weight reduction of 1 kg is associated with a lowering of systolic and diastolic BP by approximately 1 mmHg.[15]

Cigarette smoking

- Though cigarette smoking and hypertension are the two most important risk factors of vascular disease, the interaction between them is complex. Cigarette

smoking may increase BP acutely, but the long-term effect of smoking on BP is less certain.
- Although smoking cessation is unlikely to reduce BP on its own, hypertensive patients should be strongly encouraged to cease smoking so as to improve their cardiovascular health.

Pharmacological Treatment

- In addition to lifestyle changes, the majority of patients require pharmacotherapy to achieve optimum BP control. The benefits of antihypertensive drugs for prevention of cardiovascular mortality and morbidity are well established.[16] There is controversy about which antihypertensive agent should be used as first-line treatment.
- Current CSANZ guidelines[4] recommend that, for a patient with uncomplicated hypertension, angiotensin-converting enzyme (ACE) inhibitors or angiotensin receptor blockers, calcium channel blockers and thiazide diuretics are all suitable first-line antihypertensive drugs, either as a monotherapy or in combination, unless they are contraindicated for other reasons (Table 14.3).
- The choice of drugs should be influenced by the age, ethnicity, race and other clinical characteristics, including co-existing medical conditions of the patient (Tables 14.4 and 14.5).

David has been self-monitoring his BP regularly and has quit smoking. Despite his taking 5 mg of perindopril, he continues to have BP above the target range. His initial

TABLE 14.3
Major Considerations

Drugs	Contraindications
Beta-blockers	Asthma, peripheral vascular disease
Beta-blockers/non-dihydropyridines calcium channel blockers (verapamil, diltiazem)	High-grade sinoatrial or atrioventricular block, significant bradycardia (heart rate <60/min)
Calcium channel blockers (especially non-dihydropyridines)	Heart failure due to systolic dysfunction
Diuretics	Gout
ACE inhibitors/angiotensin receptor blocker	Pregnancy, hyperkalaemia (K+ >5.5 mmol/L), bilateral renal artery stenosis

TABLE 14.4
Co-Existing Conditions

Indications	Drugs
Angina	Beta-blockers, calcium channel blockers
Atrial fibrillation, supraventricular tachycardia	Beta-blockers, non-dihydropyridines calcium channel blockers
Heart failure	ACE inhibitors, angiotensin receptor blockers, beta-blockers
Diabetes, proteinuria	ACE inhibitors, angiotensin receptor blockers
Benign prostatic hypertrophy	Alpha-blockers
Peripheral vascular disease	Calcium channel blockers

investigations, including renal function tests and electrolytes, have been unremarkable. David's lipid profile showed his total cholesterol is 4.9 mmol/L, HDL cholesterol 1.06 mmol/L, LDL cholesterol 2.6 mmol/L and the ratio of total cholesterol to HDL cholesterol is 4.6.

His chest x-ray showed slight cardiomegaly but he had no other evidence of heart failure or other abnormalities. Subsequent echocardiography confirmed evidence of mild, concentric left ventricular hypertrophy with preserved systolic function.

He was prescribed a combination of perindopril 5 mg and amlodipine 5 mg daily and was encouraged to continue with a healthy active lifestyle.

Mono Therapy vs Combination Treatment

The aggregate of available data suggests that at least 75% of patients require combination therapy to achieve contemporary blood pressure targets.[17]

- In the Antihypertensive and Lipid-Lowering Treatment to Prevent Heart Attack Trial (ALLHAT), only 26% patients achieved the target BP with monotherapy.[18]
- Monotherapy may be appropriate in low-risk patients with systolic BP <150 mmHg. It is unlikely to be effective in a patient who would require a BP reduction of more than 20 mmHg to achieve target.
- Initial combination therapy is more effective than monotherapy at lowering BP. The combination of medications from different drug groups works on different targets through different mechanisms to achieve optimum BP control. Combination treatment

has been found to be better tolerated, and patients taking single-tablet combination treatment are more likely to be adherent in the long term. Current ESC guidelines recommend combination treatment for most hypertensive patients as initial therapy.

- A combination of an ACE inhibitor (ACEI), or angiotensin receptor blocker (ARB), with a calcium channel blocker (CCB) or thiazide-like diuretic is the preferred initial therapy for most patients. For those requiring three drugs, a combination of an ACE inhibitor, or ARB, with a CCB and a thiazide-like diuretic should be used (Box 14.1).
- Beta-blockers should be used when there is a specific indication for their use, for example in angina, following myocardial infarction, in left ventricular systolic dysfunction, or in the presence of ventricular or supraventricular arrhythmias.[5]
- Spironolactone is indicated as the fourth line of drug (after ACEI/ARB+CCB+thiazide or thiazide-like diuretics) for the treatment of resistant hypertension, unless the patient has significant renal impairment or hyperkalaemia.

Target Blood Pressure

- The 2018 ESC/ESH HTN guidelines recommend that the first objective of treatment should be to lower BP to <140/90 mmHg in all patients, including independent older patients who can tolerate treatment.
- The aim should also be to target BP to 130/80 mmHg for most patients, if tolerated. Even-lower office systolic BP levels (<130 mmHg) should be considered in patients aged <65 years but not in patients aged 65 years or more. Similar BP targets are recommended for patients with diabetes.
- In patients <65 years, it is recommended that systolic BP should be lowered to a range of 120–129 mmHg in most patients, and in older patients the target systolic BP should be between 130 and 139 mmHg.[5]
- A meta-analysis assessing the effects of intensive BP lowering on cardiovascular and renal outcomes involving 44,989 patients from 19 trials showed that patients in the more-intensive BP-lowering treatment group had a mean BP of 133/76 mmHg, compared with 140/81 mmHg in the less-intensive treatment group. Intensive BP-lowering treatment achieved 14% relative risk reduction for major cardiovascular events, 13% reduction of myocardial infarction, 22% reduction of stroke and 10% reduction in albuminuria.[19]
- A randomised trial of intensive versus standard BP control among patients at high risk of cardiovascular events, but without diabetes, (the SPRINT trial) showed

TABLE 14.5
Commonly Used Antihypertensive Drugs and Usual Dosages

Drugs that work on renin–angiotensin system	• Angiotensin-converting enzyme inhibitors	Ramipril	2.5–10 mg/day
		Perindopril	4–8 mg/day
		Fosinopril	10–40 mg/day
		Lisinopril	10–40 mg/day
		Quinapril	10–40 mg/day
		Captopril	12.5–100 mg twice daily
	• Angiotensin receptor blockers	Candesartan	8–32 mg/day
		Irbesartan	150–300 mg/day
		Olmesartan	20–40 mg/day
		Telmisartan	40–80 mg/day
		Valsartan	80–320 mg/day
		Losartan	50–100 mg/day
Calcium channel blockers	• Dihydropyridine	Amlodipine	5–10 mg/day
		Felodipine	5–10 mg/day
		Nifedipine	30–90 mg/day
		Lercanidipine	10–20 mg/day
	• Non-dihydropyridines	Diltiazem	120–360 mg/day
		Verapamil	120–480 mg/day
Beta-blockers	• Non-selective • Selective	Propranolol	40–80 mg twice daily
		Carvedilol	12.5–25 mg twice daily
		Atenolol	50–100 mg daily
		Metoprolol	50–100 mg twice daily
		Bisoprolol	2.5–10 mg daily
Alpha-blockers		Prazosin	0.5 mg twice daily. Max 20 mg daily
Vasodilators		Hydralazine	Initially 25–50 mg twice daily
		Minoxidil	5–40 mg daily
Diuretics	• Loop diuretics (generally not recommended unless volume overloaded)	Frusemide	Usually 40–80 mg daily
	• Potassium-sparing diuretics • Thiazide or thiazide like diuretics	Spironolactone	50–100 mg daily.
		Hydrochlorothiazide	12.5–50 mg daily
		Chlortalidone	12.5–25 mg daily
		Indapamide	1.5–2.5 mg daily
Central alpha-agonists		Methyldopa	250 mg twice daily; max 3 g/day
		Clonidine	50–100 µg, 2–3 times daily

that targeting systolic BP to less than 120 mmHg, as compared with less than 140 mmHg, produced a 43% relative risk reduction of cardiovascular mortality and a 27% relative risk reduction for all-cause mortality. The incidence of adverse events, including hypotension, syncope, electrolyte abnormalities and acute or chronic kidney injury episodes, was significantly higher in the aggressive-BP-control group.

• Unlike previous hypertension trials, the SPRINT trial used unattended automatic BP measurement, which may have resulted in lower values relative to conventional office BP measurement, owing to absence of a white coat effect.[20]

Resistant Hypertension

• Resistant hypertension is defined as suboptimal BP control despite treatment with at least three BP-lowering drugs of different classes, including a diuretic. Typically, a patient with resistant hypertension is already on a renin-acting agent (an ACE inhibitor or

> **BOX 14.1**
> **Drugs Treatment Strategy for Uncomplicated Hypertension**
>
> - In addition to lifestyle changes, consider monotherapy in low-risk hypertensive patients with systolic BP <150 mmHg.
> - If BP is inadequately controlled and, unless there is a specific indication for a particular antihypertensive agent, consider an ACEI/ARB+dihydropyridine CCB or a thiazide-type diuretic (if the patient is over 65 years old).
> - If BP is inadequately controlled, consider a combination of an ACEI/ARB+dihydropyridine CCB and a thiazide or thiazide-type diuretic.
> - For resistant hypertension, unless contraindicated, consider adding spironolactone.

ACEI=angiotensin-converting enzyme inhibitor; ARB=angiotensin receptor blocker; BP=blood pressure; CCB=calcium channel blocker.

an angiotensin receptor blocker), a calcium channel blocker and a thiazide-like diuretic and then requires a fourth-line therapy to control BP adequately.

- The prevalence of resistance hypertension varies significantly, depending on the patient population studied. In the ALLHAT[18] trial, 12.7% patients had uncontrolled BP despite treatment with at least three or more antihypertensive medications.
- PATHWAY-2 was a randomised, double-blind trial to determine the role of different antihypertensive (fourth-line) drugs in the optimal treatment of resistant hypertension, where patients were randomised to spironolactone (aldosterone antagonist), bisoprolol (beta-blocker), doxazosin (alpha-1 adrenergic receptor blocker) and placebo. The study showed that spironolactone, 25–50 mg daily, was the most effective BP-lowering treatment for patients with resistant hypertension and was well tolerated.[21]

Device-Based Therapy for Hypertension

- The sympathetic nervous system plays an important role in vascular resistance, renin release and sodium reabsorption. Activation of the renal sympathetic nerves is key to the pathogenesis of hypertension. Surgical sympathectomy has been used effectively as a treatment of severe hypertension in the past. Clinical evidence for the role of catheter-based renal denervation in resistant hypertension is conflicting. Initial trials showed promising results, but subsequently a sham-controlled randomised trial, SIMPLICITY

HTN-3, showed that renal denervation was not superior to drug therapy.[22]

- At this stage the use of device-based therapies is not recommended for the routine treatment of hypertension, unless in the context of clinical studies.[23]

Whom to Refer to a Specialist

- Younger patients (<40 years) with grade 2 hypertension or suspected secondary hypertension.
- Patients with resistant hypertension (hypertension despite treatment with three different drugs, including a diuretic).
- Patients with sudden onset of hypertension when previous BP control has been adequate.

David has been taking his BP at home (though not too often). Readings have been between 120 and 135 systolic and between 70 and 75 diastolic.

He has had no ill effects from the treatment apart from some mild ankle oedema in hot weather.

He is pleased that his health improved and the future risk of cardiovascular disease has been reduced and is happy to continue his treatment.

REFERENCES

1. Australian Bureau of Statistics. *Australian Health Survey 2014/15.* https://www.abs.gov.au.
2. Lewington S, Clarke R, Qizilbash N, Peto R, Collins R, Prospective Studies Collaboration. Age-specific relevance of usual blood pressure to vascular mortality: a meta-analysis of individual data for one million adults in 61 prospective studies. *Lancet* 2002;**360**:1903–13.
3. Ettehad D, Emdin CA, Kiran A, Anderson SG, Callender T, Emberson J, et al. Blood pressure lowering for prevention of cardiovascular disease and death: a systematic review and meta-analysis. *Lancet* 2016;**387**(10022):957–67.
4. Anderson C, Arnolda L, Cowley D, Dowden J, Gabb G, Golledge J, et al. National Heart Foundation hypertension guideline – 2016. *Heart Lung Circ* 2016;**25**:S18. https://www.heartfoundation.org.au/for-professionals/clinical-information/hypertension.
5. Williams B, Mancia G, Spiering W, Rosei EA, Azizi M, Burnier M, et al; ESC Scientific Document Group. 2018 ESC/ESH Guidelines for the management of arterial hypertension: the Task Force for the management of arterial hypertension of the European Society of Cardiology (ESC) and the European Society of Hypertension (ESH). *Eur Heart J* 2018;**39**(33):3021–104.
6. Whelton PK, Carey RM, Aronow WS, Casey DE Jr, Collins KJ, Dennison Himmelfarb C, et al. 2017 ACC/AHA: a guideline for the prevention, detection, evaluation, and management of high blood pressure in adults: a report of the American College of Cardiology/American Heart

Association Task Force on Clinical Practice Guidelines. *Hypertension* 2018;**71**(6):e13–115.

7. Weber MA, Schiffrin EL, White WB, Mann S, Lindholm LH, Kenerson JG, et al; Clinical Practice Guidelines for the Management of Hypertension in the Community. A Statement by the American Society of Hypertension and the International Society of Hypertension. *J Clin Hypertens* 2014;**16**(1):14–26.

8. Dickinson HO, Mason JM, Nicolson DJ, Campbell F, Beyer FR, Cook JV, et al. Lifestyle interventions to reduce raised blood pressure: a systematic review of randomized controlled trials. *J Hypertens* 2006;**24**:215–33.

9. Cornelissen VA, Buys R, Smart NA. Endurance exercise beneficially affects ambulatory blood pressure: a systematic review and meta-analysis. *J Hypertens* 2013;**31**:639.

10. Moore TJ, Conlin PR, Ard J, Svetkey LP. DASH (Dietary Approaches to Stop Hypertension) diet is effective treatment for stage 1 isolated systolic hypertension. *Hypertension* 2001;**38**:155–8.

11. Domenech M, Roman P, Lapetra J, Garcia de la Corte FJ, Sala-Vila A, de la Torre R, et al. Mediterranean diet reduces 24-hour ambulatory blood pressure, blood glucose, and lipids: one-year randomized, clinical trial. *Hypertension* 2014;**64**:69–76.

12. Graudal NA, Hubeck-Graudal T, Jurgens G. Effects of low sodium diet versus high sodium diet on blood pressure, renin, aldosterone, catecholamines, cholesterol, and triglyceride (Cochrane Review). *Am J Hypertens* 2012;**25**(1):1–15.

13. National Heart Foundation of Australia. *Summary of evidence statement on the relationship between dietary electrolytes and cardiovascular disease.* NHFA; 2006.

14. Taylor B, Irving HM, Baliunas D, Roerecke M, Patra J, Mohapatra S, et al. Alcohol and hypertension: gender differences in dose–response relationships determined through systematic review and meta-analysis. *Addiction* 2009;**104**(12):1981–90.

15. Neter JE, Stam BE, Kok FJ, Grobbee DE, Geleijnse JM. Influence of weight reduction on blood pressure: a meta-analysis of randomized controlled trials. *Hypertension* 2003;**42**:878–84.

16. Turnbull F, Blood Pressure Lowering Treatment Trialists' Collaboration. Effects of different blood-pressure-lowering regimens on major cardiovascular events: results of prospectively-designed overviews of randomised trials. *Lancet* 2003;**362**:1527.

17. Gradman AH, Basile JN, Carter BL, Bakris GL. Combination therapy in hypertension. *J Clin Hypertens (Greenwich)* 2011;**13**(3):146–54.

18. Muntner P, Davis BR, Cushman WC, Bangalore S, Calhoun DA, Pressel SL, et al; ALLHAT Collaborative Research Group. Treatment-resistant hypertension and the incidence of cardiovascular disease and end-stage renal disease: results from the Antihypertensive and Lipid-Lowering Treatment to Prevent Heart Attack Trial (ALLHAT). *Hypertension* 2014;**64**:1012–21.

19. Xie X, Atkins E, Lv J, Bennett A, Neal B, Ninomiya T, et al. Effects of intensive blood pressure lowering on cardiovascular and renal outcomes: updated systematic review and meta-analysis. *Lancet* 2016;**387**(10017):435–43.

20. Wright JT Jr, Williamson JD, Whelton PK, Snyder JK, Sink KM, Rocco MV, et al. A randomized trial of intensive versus standard blood-pressure control. *N Engl J Med* 2015;**373**(22):2103–16.

21. Williams B, MacDonald TM, Morant S, Webb DJ, Sever P, McInnes G, et al; British Hypertension Society's PATHWAY Studies Group. Spironolactone versus placebo, bisoprolol, and doxazosin to determine the optimal treatment for drug-resistant hypertension (PATHWAY-2): a randomised, double-blind, crossover trial. *Lancet* 2015;**386**(10008):2059–68.

22. Bhatt DL, Kandzari DE, O'Neill WW, D'Agostino R, Flack JM, Katzen BT, et al. SYMPLICITY HTN-3 Investigators. A controlled trial of renal denervation for resistant hypertension. *N Engl J Med* 2014;**370**:1393–401.

23. Williams B, Mancia G, Spiering W, Agabiti Rosei E, Azizi M, Burnier M, et al; ESC Scientific Document Group. 2018 ESC/ESH Guidelines for the management of arterial hypertension. *Eur Heart J* 2018;**39**(33):3021–104.

CHAPTER 15

Heart Failure

CASE 18 SCENARIO: ROBERT WITH DYSPNOEA

Forty-six-year-old Robert presented to the hospital with increasing dyspnoea for the last 2 weeks. He has found it difficult to lie flat in bed and has been waking up frequently feeling breathless. For the last few nights he has been sleeping on a recliner. He also has a dry cough and has felt extremely tired. He has a previous history of type II diabetes, for which he takes metformin.

Robert had an anterior myocardial infarction 6 weeks previously while on holiday and presented to a rural hospital 3 days after the initial episode of chest pain. He was transferred to a tertiary hospital, when coronary angiography showed an 80% stenosis of the proximal left anterior descending artery that was stented.

His echocardiogram performed while he was in hospital showed left ventricular anterior wall akinesia with an ejection fraction of 30%.

He has no past history of asthma. He is a lifelong non-smoker.

His current medications include aspirin 100 mg/day, ticagrelor 90 mg twice daily, bisoprolol 2.5 mg daily, atorvastatin 40 mg daily and ramipril 2.5 mg daily.

Robert's physical examination revealed:
- a regular pulse with a rate of 96/minute
- oxygen saturation of 93% on room air
- blood pressure of 123/78 mmHg
- elevation of the jugular venous pressure to 6 cm
- a third heart sound and a pansystolic murmur
- a positive hepatojugular reflux test; and
- he also has bilateral crackles in the lung bases, scattered wheezes and mild pitting oedema in both ankles.

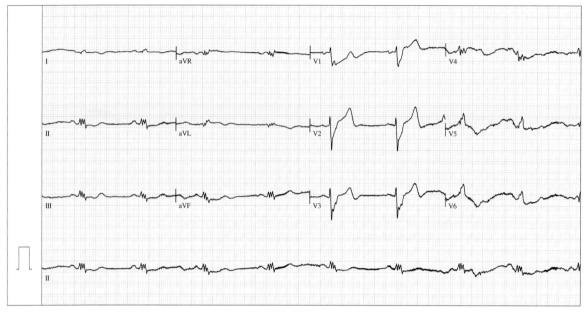

FIG. 15.1 ECG showing sinus rhythm with (wide QRS complex) left bundle branch block (pre-CRT).

The examination findings and history were consistent with a diagnosis of heart failure.

Questions
1. *What is heart failure?*
2. *How would you investigate and manage Robert?*
3. *Please describe the role of pharmacotherapy in heart failure.*

His ECG showed sinus rhythm with left bundle branch block, which was unchanged from the previous ECG (Fig. 15.1).

His urgent chest x-ray showed cardiomegaly and evidence of pulmonary oedema.

Robert had an echocardiogram, which looked the same as his previous one. The ejection fraction was again 30% (Fig. 15.2). There was segmental left ventricular dysfunction. He also had moderate, functional mitral regurgitation. His echocardiographic features were consistent with ischaemic cardiomyopathy.

DEFINITION OF HEART FAILURE
- Heart failure is a complex clinical syndrome that results from any structural or functional impairment of ventricular filling or ejection of blood.
- The clinical syndrome of heart failure may result from disorders of the pericardium, myocardium, endocardium, heart valves or great vessels, or from certain metabolic abnormalities, but most patients with HF have symptoms due to impaired left ventricular (LV) myocardial function.[1]

SYMPTOMS OF HEART FAILURE
- Heart failure is a clinical syndrome characterised by typical symptoms that may be accompanied by signs caused by a structural or functional cardiac abnormality, or both, resulting in a reduced cardiac output with or without elevated intracardiac pressures at rest or during stress.[2]
- The typical symptoms of heart failure include:
  - exertional dyspnoea
  - orthopnoea
  - paroxysmal nocturnal dyspnoea
  - ankle swelling
  - fatigue
  - weakness.
- Nocturnal dry cough also may be a feature of heart failure and can be can be mistakenly diagnosed as asthma, gastrointestinal reflux or ACE inhibitor-induced cough.

INCIDENCE AND PREVALENCE OF HEART FAILURE
With better management strategy in treatment and prevention of coronary artery disease and the early

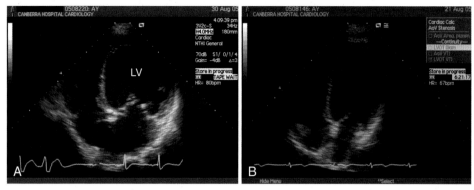

FIG. 15.2 Echocardiography in **(A)** a patient with dilated cardiomyopathy showing enlarged, dilated, globular left ventricle (LV) and **(B)** normal heart.

revascularisation of acute coronary syndrome patients, the incidence of age-adjusted new HF diagnosis is stable or decreasing. Despite that, due to improvement of effective anti-failure therapy, there is a worldwide increase in HF prevalence (the number of cases with HF diagnosis who are alive). In Australia, in 2014, it was estimated that there were 480,000 people aged 18 years or more with HF, representing 2.1% of the total adult population.[3]

The lifetime risk of developing HF for women and men at age 55 years is 29% and 33% respectively.[4]

PATHOGENESIS

- Heart failure is associated with complex neuro-hormonal changes including activation of the renin–angiotensin–aldosterone axis and the sympathetic nervous system.
- Initially these changes may be helpful in maintaining blood pressure and cardiac output, but ultimately they become counterproductive. This is partly as a result of increased cardiac fibrosis resulting from these maladaptive changes. Understanding the neuro-hormonal changes is very important in the treatment of HF.

CAUSES OF HEART FAILURE

Nearly any form of heart disease may ultimately lead to HF:

- Heart failure risk factors vary substantially among world regions. Coronary artery disease and prior myocardial infarction account for approximately two-thirds of systolic HF cases.[5]

- Ischaemic heart disease – is a risk factor for HF in >50% of patients in Western high-income and Eastern and Central European regions, 30%–40% in East Asia, Asia-Pacific high-income and Latin American and Caribbean regions, and <10% in sub-Saharan Africa.[6]
- Hypertension – may contribute to HF via increased afterload and acceleration of coronary artery disease. Hypertension is a major risk factor for the development of both heart failure due to reduced systolic function (HFrEF) and heart failure with preserved systolic function (HFpEF). Hypertension is a commonly reported risk factor in all regions, with an approximately 17% or more crude prevalence among HF cases.[6]
- Idiopathic dilated cardiomyopathy – patients tend to be younger, and at least 30% of cases appear to be familial. Idiopathic dilated cardiomyopathy is present in approximately 5%–10% of new cases of HF.[7]
- Valvular heart disease – including congenital and acquired valvular disease.
- Infiltrative disease – including amyloidosis, sarcoidosis and haemochromatosis.
- Chronic alcoholism – is one of the most important causes of cardiomyopathy and HF. Alcoholic cardiomyopathy most commonly occurs in men 30–55 years of age who have been heavy consumers of alcohol for >10 years.[8]
- Several cytotoxic antineoplastic drugs – especially the anthracyclines, monoclonal antibody trastuzumab (Herceptin), high-dose cyclophosphamide, taxoids, mitomycin-C, 5-fluorouracil and the interferons are cardiotoxic and can lead to cardiomyopathy and HF.[9]

- Infectious myocarditis – especially coxsackie B virus and HIV.
- Tachycardia-related cardiomyopathy – should be considered in all patients with heart failure due to systolic dysfunction of uncertain origin and who have atrial flutter/fibrillation with a rapid ventricular rate or frequent ventricular ectopic beats with high ectopic load.
- Endocrine disorders – hypothyroidism, hyper-thyroidism.
- Peripartum cardiomyopathy – is a disease of unknown cause in which LV dysfunction occurs during the last trimester of pregnancy or the early puerperium.
- Stress cardiomyopathy (takotsubo cardiomyopathy) – is characterised by acute reversible LV dysfunction in the absence of significant coronary artery disease. It is frequently triggered by acute emotional or physical stress.

CLASSIFICATION OF HEART FAILURE

The primary classification of heart failure is currently based on LV ejection fraction.

Heart Failure With Reduced Systolic Function

Heart failure with reduced ejection fraction (HFrEF) is defined as the presence of clinical symptoms with or without signs of heart failure, and an ejection fraction of less than 50%.

Heart Failure With Preserved Systolic Function

- Heart failure with preserved ejection fraction (HFpEF) is a clinical syndrome in which patients have symptoms with or without signs of heart failure (HF) and a left ventricular ejection fraction (LVEF) ≥50%.[2]
- Various studies estimate that as many as 40%–60% of patients with HF have a normal LVEF.[10]
- There are no significant differences between the HFrEF and HFpEF groups in post-discharge mortality or rehospitalisation. Similarly, there is no significant difference in death or rehospitalisation from any cause.[11]
- Patients with HFpEF are older and more likely to be female and commonly have a history of hypertension and atrial fibrillation.[11]
- Differentiation between systolic and diastolic heart failure can be difficult on the basis of history, physical examination, ECG or chest x-ray (CXR) alone.

DIAGNOSTIC CRITERIA FOR HEART FAILURE WITH PRESERVED SYSTOLIC FUNCTION

- Presence of symptoms or signs of heart failure, or both.
- Presence of normal or near normal LV systolic function (LVEF >50%).
- Elevated level of natriuretic peptides.
- Evidence of relevant structural heart disease (left ventricular hypertrophy or left atrial enlargement), or
- Diastolic dysfunction – documented high left-sided intracavity filling pressure, measured invasively or by echocardiography. At least three of the following:
  - mitral annular velocity (septal) e' <7 cm/s, lateral e' <10 cm/s.
  - mitral valve E/e' ratio >14.
  - left atrial volume index >34 mL/m^2
  - tricuspid valve regurgitation velocity >2.8 m/s.[2,12]

HEART FAILURE WITH PRESERVED SYSTOLIC FUNCTION – DIFFERENTIAL DIAGNOSIS

Heart failure with preserved systolic function is quite often a diagnosis of exclusion. The differential diagnosis that needs to be considered includes:

- **cardiac causes:** heart failure with reduced systolic function, hypertrophic cardiomyopathy, constrictive pericarditis, chronic effusive pericarditis, valvular heart disease, intracardiac shunt
- **respiratory causes:** chronic obstructive lung disease, interstitial lung disease, chronic thromboembolic disease, pulmonary hypertension
- **other causes:** chronic liver disease, nephrotic syndrome, anaemia, thyroid disease.

INVESTIGATING HEART FAILURE

Basic investigations of suspected heart failure include:

- non-invasive measurement of oxygen saturation
- serum electrolytes
- renal function (may be abnormal due to low renal perfusion, associated renovascular disease or treatment with diuretics, ACE inhibitors, etc.)
- liver function (often abnormal due to congestion)
- full blood count (to exclude anaemia as a cause of heart failure)
- thyroid function tests (to exclude thyrotoxicosis)
- arterial blood gases and D-dimer (to exclude pulmonary embolism as a cause of dyspnoea).

Troponin measurement may be helpful in selective cases. Troponin elevation in patients with heart failure is relatively common. In an analysis of the ADHERE (Acute Decompensated Heart Failure National Registry) study, 75% of patients hospitalised with acute HF (*n*=67,924) had detectable levels of troponin.[13] The mechanism of underlying troponin release in patients with HF is not clear and is probably multifactorial. Though ischaemia is an important cause of HF, many patients in HF with troponin elevation may not have underlying obstructive coronary artery disease. Numerous studies have demonstrated the association between elevated troponin and adverse clinical outcomes in patients with HF. Although elevated troponins have prognostic value in HF, they are poor diagnostic markers for an ischaemic versus non-ischaemic aetiology of HF.[14] (See also Chapter 10.)

A 12-lead ECG in a patient with HF is rarely completely normal. Common abnormalities include atrial fibrillation, previous myocardial infarction, left ventricular hypertrophy, bundle branch block and axis deviation. The ECG is sensitive but very non-specific; a normal ECG virtually rules out HF.[15]

Chest X-ray

In the acute setting a CXR may show pulmonary venous congestion in a patient with heart failure. It may also show cardiomegaly, although a patient with significant left ventricular dysfunction may present without cardiomegaly on the CXR. The CXR is also useful in identifying alternative pulmonary or other diseases that could explain the patient's symptoms and signs (Fig. 15.3).

Echocardiogram

The echocardiogram is the most important test in suspected heart failure. It provides information on ventricular size and systolic function, as well as the presence of scars related to previous myocardial infarction. Echocardiography is also very useful in determining whether the underlying aetiology has an ischaemic or non-ischaemic basis. In addition, the detection of other structural heart disease, including valvular abnormalities, raised pulmonary artery pressures and the presence or absence of pericardial disease, may be of use in guiding therapy as well as assisting in the diagnosis. Tissue Doppler imaging is of particular importance in diagnosing heart failure with preserved systolic function.

B-type Natriuretic Peptides[12]

- B-type natriuretic peptides (BNPs) are vasoactive peptides that result in natriuresis, diuresis and vasodilation. They may be viewed as the body's endogenous defence against hypervolaemia and hypertension. BNP is a propeptide and is released from myocytes in response to increased wall tension.
- The propeptide (proBNP) is released into the circulation and then cleaved into biologically active BNP and its biologically inactive NT fragment (NT proBNP).
- The high negative predictive value of BNP tests is particularly helpful for ruling out heart failure. However, increases in BNP levels may be caused by intrinsic cardiac dysfunction or may be secondary to other causes such as pulmonary or renal disease.
- For heart failure patients taking valsartan / sacubitril (Entresto), NT proBNP (rather than plain BNP) must

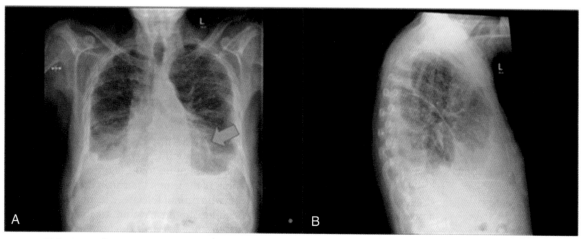

FIG. 15.3 Chest x-ray posteroanterior **(A)** and lateral view **(B)** from a patient with congestive heart failure, and bilateral pleural effusion due to constrictive pericarditis. Arrow shows calcified pericardium.

be for assessment of HF, as degradation of BNP is blocked by Entresto, causing 'falsely high' levels. The N-terminal component is unaffected.

MANAGEMENT OF HEART FAILURE WITH REDUCED SYSTOLIC FUNCTION
Non-pharmacological Management

This includes:
- regular physical activity
- nutrition
- salt and water restriction
- alcohol abstinence
- smoking cessation
- avoidance of medications that can precipitate heart failure (Table 15.1).

Physical activity has been shown to improve functional capacity, symptoms and neurohormonal abnormalities. Patients should be encouraged to walk daily for 30 minutes/day for 5 days a week.

TABLE 15.1
Common Medications That May Exacerbate Heart Failure

Class	Drugs
Non-steroidal anti-inflammatory agents	Ibuprofen, indomethacin, diclofenac
COX-2 inhibitors	Celecoxib
Non-dihydropyridine calcium channel blockers	Diltiazem, verapamil
Centrally acting alpha-adrenergic medications	Moxonidine
Type I antiarrhythmic drugs	Flecainide, disopyramide and quinidine
Glitazone	Pioglitazone, rosiglitazone
Dipeptidyl peptidase-4 inhibitors	Saxagliptin, sitagliptin
Antipsychotics	Clozapine
HER2 receptor antagonist	Trastuzumab (Herceptin)
Anthracyline chemotherapeutic agents	Doxorubicin, daunorubicin, epirubicin, idarubicin, mitoxantrone
Alkylating agents	Cyclophosphamide, ifosfamide
Other agents	Anabolic steroids, chloroquine, etanercept

Pharmacological Management

The pharmacological management of heart failure is based on an understanding of the two main pathophysiological mechanisms and consists of:
1. inhibition of the renin–angiotensin–aldosterone system (RAAS)
2. inhibition of the sympathetic nervous system.

Inhibition of the renin–angiotensin–aldosterone system

- The RAAS is activated by renal hypoperfusion and sympathetic activation. The key product of this cascade is angiotensin II. Angiotensin II has widespread haemodynamic and vascular effects on the cardiovascular system that are initially compensatory but subsequently exacerbate the heart failure syndrome. Angiotensin II activates AT1 receptors, leading to a range of effects including vasoconstriction, cellular proliferation, and pro-oxidative and pro-inflammatory actions.
- Both ACE inhibitors and angiotensin receptor blockers (ARBs) attenuate the effects of angiotensin II, but through different mechanisms – ACE inhibitors reduce the synthesis of angiotensin II, whereas ARBs bind to AT receptors to block their activation.[16]
- ACE inhibitors also increase bradykinin levels, leading to additional cardiovascular effects including vasodilation.
- ACE inhibitors and ARBs are the drugs most commonly used to provide therapeutic modulation of angiotensin II. Important trials of inhibition of the renin–angiotensin–aldosterone system are summarised in Table 15.2.

Angiotensin-converting enzyme inhibitors

- ACE inhibitors are the first-line treatment in patients with poor left ventricular systolic function (LVEF <40%). There is clear evidence that these drugs prolong survival, reduce progression of heart failure and improve quality of life. Every patient with HF due to systolic dysfunction should be on an ACE inhibitor unless contraindicated.[17]
- Common side effects of ACE inhibitors include a dry cough in 5%–10% cases, hyperkalaemia due to decreased aldosterone secretion, angioedema (fatal in some cases) in up to 0.2% of patients and renal dysgenesis of the fetus if the drug is used in pregnancy.
- Patients who cannot tolerate ACE inhibitors because of coughing should have an angiotensin receptor blocker. In some selected patients the addition of an ARB to an ACE inhibitor can be considered, but there is a risk of hyperkalaemia and of precipitating an

TABLE 15.2
Important Trials of Inhibition of the Renin–Angiotensin–Aldosterone System

Trial Name	Drug	Dosage	Criteria	Result
CONSENSUS	Enalapril	2.5–40 mg per day	Severe congestive HF (NYHA functional class IV)	A reduction of 40% ($P=0.002$) in mortality in the enalapril group at the end of 6 months
V-HeFT II	Enalapril vs hydralazine/ isosorbide-dinitrate	300 mg of hydralazine plus 160 mg of isosorbide dinitrate daily vs enalapril 20 mg daily	Cardiothoracic ratio ≥0.55 on CXR, LV end-diastolic diameter >2.7 cm/m^2 or ejection fraction <45% as determined with radionuclide methods and reduced exercise tolerance	V-HeFT II demonstrated that enalapril had a more favorable effect on 2-year survival than a combination of hydralazine plus isosorbide dinitrate
SOLVD	Enalapril	2.5–20 mg per day	NYHA Class II to III HF and EF <35%	16% fewer deaths in the enalapril group, primarily deaths attributed to progressive HF, and 26% fewer hospitalisations
Val-HeFT	Valsartan	160 mg of valsartan or placebo twice daily	Heart failure (Class II to IV) with ejection fraction of <40%, and LV dilation and receiving standard treatment	13.2% reduction in combined end point of mortality and morbidity, and improved clinical signs and symptoms of HF
CHARM-Alternative trial	Candesartan	Starting dose was 4–8 mg once daily, and target dose of 32 mg once daily	Patients with LV dysfunction, EF 40% or less Intolerant to ACEIs	23% relative risk reduction in cardiovascular mortality or hospital admission for HF with candesartan
RALES	Spironolactone	25–50 mg once daily	Class III and IV HF patients with systolic dysfunction, EF ≥35%	30% reduction in the relative risk ($P<0.001$) of all-cause mortality
EPHESUS	Eplerenone	25 mg daily initially, titrated to a maximum of 50 mg daily	3–14 days after acute myocardial infarction, EF 40% or less and HF	15% relative risk reduction in all-cause mortality and a 13% risk reduction in cardiovascular mortality or hospitalisation for cardiovascular events
PARADIGM-HF	Sacubitril/ valsartan (Entresto)	Entresto 97/103 mg twice daily vs enalapril 10 mg twice daily	NYHA class II–IV; systolic dysfunction with left ventricular EF ≤40%	Entresto reduced the risk of cardiovascular death by 20% and heart failure hospitalisation by 21%

ACEI=angiotensin-converting enzyme inhibitor; CXR=chest x-ray; EF=ejection fraction; HF=heart failure; LV=left ventricle; NYHA=New York Heart Association.

(Data from: CONSENSUS Trial Study Group. Effects of enalapril on mortality in severe congestive heart failure. Results of the Cooperative North Scandinavian Enalapril Survival Study (CONSENSUS). *N Engl J Med* 1987;316(23):1429–35; Cohn JN, Johnson G, Ziesche S, Cobb F, Francis G, Tristani F, et al. A comparison of enalapril with hydralazine-isosorbide dinitrate in the treatment of chronic congestive heart failure. *N Engl J Med* 1991;325:303–10; SOLVD Investigators, Yusuf S, Pitt B, Davis CE, Hood WB, Cohn JN. Effect of enalapril on survival in patients with reduced left ventricular ejection fractions and congestive heart failure. *N Engl J Med* 1991;325:293; Cohn JN, Tognoni G; Valsartan Heart Failure Trial Investigators. A randomized trial of the angiotensin-receptor blocker valsartan in chronic heart failure. *N Engl J Med* 2001;345:1667–75; Granger CB, McMurray JJ, Yusuf S, Held P, Michelson EL, Olofsson B, et al. Effects of candesartan in patients with chronic heart failure and reduced left-ventricular systolic function intolerant to angiotensin-converting-enzyme inhibitors: the CHARM-Alternative trial. *Lancet* 2003;362(9386):772–6; Pitt B, Zannad F, Remme WJ, Held P, Michelson EL, Olofsson B, et al.; CHARM Investigators and Committees. The effect of spironolactone on morbidity and mortality in patients with severe heart failure. Randomized Aldactone Evaluation Study Investigators. *N Engl J Med* 1999;341:709; Pitt B, Remme W, Zannad F, Neaton J, Martinez F, Roniker B, et al; Eplerenone Post-Acute Myocardial Infarction Heart Failure Efficacy and Survival Study Investigators. Eplerenone, a selective aldosterone blocker, in patients with left ventricular dysfunction after myocardial infarction. *N Engl J Med* 2003;348:1309–21; McMurray JJV, Packer M, Desai AS, Gong J, Lefkowitz MP, Rizkala AR, et al.; PARADIGM-HF Investigators and Committees. Angiotensin–neprilysin inhibition versus enalapril in heart failure. N Engl J Med 2014;371(11):993–1004.)

acute kidney injury. Patients who cannot tolerate ACE inhibitors because of chronic kidney disease and hyperkalaemia should be considered for treatment with hydralazine and nitrates in combination.

Angiotensin II receptor blockers

- ARBs have been shown to reduce the risk of hospitalisation for heart failure and of cardiovascular death in symptomatic patients unable to tolerate an ACE inhibitor because of unacceptable side effects (usually a dry cough).
- In the Val-HeFT trial, patients with heart failure were randomly assigned to receive 160 mg of valsartan or placebo twice daily. Valsartan significantly reduced the combined end point of mortality and morbidity, and improved clinical signs and symptoms in these patients, when added to prescribed therapy.[18]
- Similarly, the CHARM trial assessed the effect of the long-acting angiotensin II type 1 receptor blocker candesartan in patients with symptomatic heart failure. Candesartan significantly reduced all-cause mortality, cardiovascular death and HF hospitalisations in patients with HF and a LVEF <40% when

added to standard therapies including ACE inhibitors, beta-blockers and an aldosterone antagonist.[19]
- An ARB is recommended in patients with heart failure with LVEF ≤40% if an ACE inhibitor is contraindicated or not tolerated, because it has been shown to decrease the combined end point of cardiovascular mortality and hospitalisation for HF.[12]

Angiotensin receptor neprilysin inhibitor (ARNI)
(Fig. 15.4)

- The natriuretic peptide system counter regulates the detrimental effects of the upregulation of RAAS that occurs in heart failure. Secretion of natriuretic peptide results in a number of responses including vasodilation, decreased sympathetic tone, increased diuresis and natriuresis, decreased release of vasopressin and aldosterone, and decreased myocardial fibrosis and hypertrophy.[20]
- Neprilysin, a neutral endopeptidase, degrades several endogenous vasoactive peptides including natriuretic peptides and bradykinin. Inhibition of neprilysin increases the levels of these substances, countering the neurohormonal overactivation seen in heart

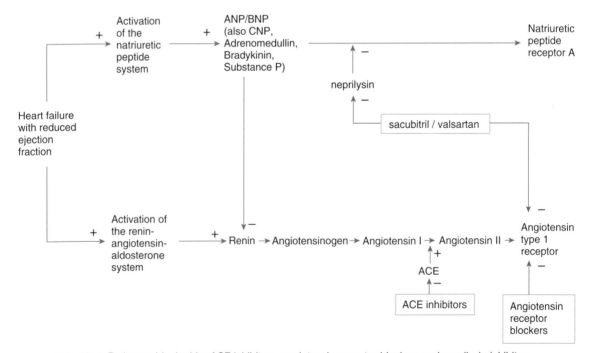

FIG. 15.4 Pathways blocked by ACE inhibitors, angiotensin receptor blockers and neprilysin inhibitors. ANP=atrial natriuretic peptide; BNP=B-type natriuretic peptide; CNP=C-type natriuretic peptide. (Reproduced with permission from Jhund PS, McMurray JJV. The neprilysin pathway in heart failure: a review and guide on the use of sacubitril/valsartan. *Heart* 2016;102:1342–7.)

failure patients, which contributes to vasoconstriction, sodium retention and maladaptive remodelling.

- In the PARADIGM-HF trial,[21] dual blockade of RAAS and the natriuretic peptide system, using a combination of the neprilysin inhibitor sacubitril and the ARB valsartan (Entresto) in patients with heart failure due to reduced ejection fraction, was more effective in reducing the risk of death from cardiovascular causes or hospitalisation for HF than was ACE inhibition with enalapril. The combination also reduced the risk of cardiovascular death by 20% and HF hospitalisation by 21%.
- In the clinical trial, the most commonly observed adverse events with sacubitril/valsartan were hypotension, hyperkalaemia and cough. Hypotension was significantly more common with sacubitril/valsartan than with enalapril (14% vs 9%).[21]
- In a patient taking an ACE inhibitor, sacubitril/valsartan (Entresto) needs to be started after a 36-hour washout period after cessation of the ACE inhibitor because of the increased risk of angioedema when the drugs are used together.

Hydralazine plus nitrates

- Hydralazine is predominantly an arteriolar dilator that reduces afterload, whereas nitrates reduce preload mainly by venous dilation. Important side effects of hydralazine include fluid retention and tachycardia. Patients on higher dosages and on prolonged therapy with hydralazine may develop drug-induced lupus syndrome. Headache is a frequently observed side effect of nitrate treatment. It can also cause significant hypotension.
- The first 5-year, multicentre Veterans Administration Cooperative Vasodilator – Heart Failure Trial (V-HeFT I) showed that treating heart failure patients with hydralazine and isosorbide dinitrate significantly reduced their mortality compared with placebo. The reduction in mortality with this combination therapy was 28% over the mean 2.3 years follow-up period.[22]
- The V-HeFT II trial demonstrated that enalapril had a more favourable effect on 2-year survival than a combination of hydralazine plus isosorbide dinitrate.[23]

Aldosterone antagonists (mineralocorticoid receptor antagonists)

- An aldosterone antagonist inhibits the aldosterone-mediated reabsorption of sodium and secretion of potassium. It also prevents myocardial and vascular fibrosis. Spironolactone and eplerenone are both mineralocorticoid receptor antagonists (MRAs) used in the treatment of heart failure.

- An aldosterone antagonist should be considered in all patients with heart failure with reduced ejection fraction (<40%), unless it is contraindicated or not tolerated, because these drugs have been shown to reduce mortality and decrease the chance of hospitalisation for HF. They are not recommended in patients with an eGFR <30 mL/min and/or a K$^+$ >5 mmol/L. Eplerenone is recommended for patients who develop systolic dysfunction early after a myocardial infarction.

Inhibition of the sympathetic nervous system

- In addition to the RAAS, the sympathetic nervous system is also intrinsic to the neuroendocrine pathophysiology of heart failure. Initially, catecholamine excess temporarily increases cardiac output via inotropic and chronotropic effects, but subsequently it exacerbates myocardial ischaemia, hypertrophy and fibrosis, and increases the likelihood of arrhythmias.[24]
- Studies showed that the degree of sympathetic activation as measured by plasma noradrenaline levels correlated with New York Heart Association (NYHA) functional capacity and prognosis, with higher levels portending a worse outcome and NYHA class.[25]
- Beta-blockers have been one of the important classes of drugs used in the treatment of heart failure because of their ability to reverse the neurohumoral effects of the sympathetic nervous system.

  Beta-blocker therapy is associated with clinically meaningful reduction in mortality and morbidity in stable euvolaemic patients with heart failure and should be offered routinely to all patients, unless contraindicated.

  Currently recommended beta-blockers for treatment of heart failure include:
  - bisoprolol
  - carvedilol
  - long-acting metoprolol, and
  - nebivolol (Table 15.3).

  Beta-blockers should be started at a low dose and gradually uptitrated at intervals of at least 2 weeks to the target dose or maximum dose that is tolerated. Hypotension or bradycardia may limit the maximum dose that can be used.

Role of Other Drugs in the Treatment of Heart Failure With Reduced Systolic Function

Diuretics

Diuretics are commonly used in patients with congestive cardiac failure to relieve symptoms (Table 15.4). Although

TABLE 15.3
Important Beta-blocker Trials in Heart Failure

Study Name	Drug	Description	Main Findings	Starting Dose (Target Dose)
CIBIS II	Bisoprolol	Heart failure; Class III–IV; EF <35%	32% decrease of mortality and hospitalisation for HF	1.25 mg daily (10 mg daily)
COPERNICUS	Carvedilol	Heart failure; Class III–IV; EF <25%	35% decrease of mortality	3.125 mg twice daily (25 mg twice daily)
CAPRICORN	Carvedilol	Recent myocardial infarction; EF <40%	23% reduction in mortality	3.125 mg twice daily (25 mg twice daily)
MERIT-HF	Metoprolol succinate	Heart failure, Class II–IV; EF <40%	34% decrease in all-cause mortality	12.5 mg daily (200 mg daily)
SENIORS	Nebivolol	Heart failure; EF< 35% in last 6 months; age >70 years	14% reduction in all-cause mortality and cardiovascular hospitalisation	1.25 mg once daily (10 mg daily)
COMET	Carvedilol vs metoprolol tartrate	Heart failure, Class II–IV; EF <35%	17% decrease in mortality with carvedilol compared with metoprolol	Carvedilol 3.125 mg twice daily/metoprolol 5 mg twice daily (25 mg twice daily/50 mg twice daily)

EF=ejection fraction.
(Data from: CIBIS II Investigators and Committees. The cardiac insufficiency bisoprolol study II (CIBIS-II): a randomised trial. *Lancet* 1999;353:9–13; Packer, M, Fowler MB, Roecker EB, Coats AJ, Katus H, Krum H, et al. Effect of carvedilol on the morbidity of patients with severe chronic heart failure: results of the carvedilol prospective randomized cumulative survival (COPERNICUS) study. *Circulation* 2002;106:2194–9; The CAPRICORN Investigators. Effect of carvedilol on outcome after myocardial infarction in patients with left-ventricular dysfunction: the CAPRICORN randomised trial. *Lancet* 2001;357(9266):1385–90; MERIT-HF Study Group. Effect of metoprolol CR/XL in chronic heart failure: metoprolol CR/XL randomised intervention trial in congestive heart failure (MERIT-HF). *Lancet* 1999;353:2001–7; Flather MD, Shibata MC, Coats AJ. Randomized trial to determine the effect of nebivolol on mortality and cardiovascular hospital admission in elderly patients with heart failure (SENIORS). *Eur Heart J* 2005;26:215–25; Carvedilol Or Metoprolol European Trial Investigators. Comparison of carvedilol and metoprolol on clinical outcomes in patients with chronic heart failure in the Carvedilol Or Metoprolol European Trial (COMET): randomised controlled trial. *Lancet* 2003;362(9377):7–13.)

TABLE 15.4
Diuretic Drugs in Heart Failure

Drug Class	Mode of Action	Drugs	Starting Dose	Maximum Dose	Side Effects
Loop diuretics	Inhibit Na/K/Cl co-transporter in the ascending limp of loop of Henle	Frusemide Bumetanide Ethacrynic acid	20–40 mg daily 0.5–1 mg daily 25—50 mg daily	600 mg 10 mg 200 mg	Hypokalaemia, hypomagnesaemia, hyperuricaemia, hypocalcaemia, gout
Thiazide-like diuretics	Inhibit Na–Cl transport at distal nephron	Hydrochlorothiazide Chlorthalidone Indapamide	12.5 mg daily 12.5 mg daily 1.25 mg daily	100 mg 50 mg 5 mg	Hyponatraemia, hypokalaemia, hypocalcaemia, hyperuricaemia, gout
Potassium-sparing diuretics	Aldosterone antagonists; block Na transport channel in the collecting tubule	Spironolactone Amiloride Triamterene	12.5–25 mg daily 2.5 mg 25 mg twice daily	200 mg 20 mg 200 mg	Hyperkalaemia, gynaecomastia

they are widely used, there are limited data on their effects on mortality and morbidity.

- Loop diuretics inhibit the $Na^+/2Cl^-/K^+$ co-transporter of the thick ascending limb of the loop of Henle, causing decreased sodium and chloride reabsorption and increased diuresis. Loop diuretics include frusemide, bumetanide and ethacrynic acid. Frusemide is by far the most common oral loop diuretic used clinically. Bumetanide may be more efficacious, owing to its increased oral bioavailability and potency.
- The dose of the diuretic for long-term use needs to be adjusted frequently depending on the patient's volume status, particularly after treatment of acute decompensation. This helps avoid dehydration, which can lead to hypotension and renal dysfunction. The aim of diuretic therapy is to achieve and maintain euvolaemia with the lowest possible dose. Patients can be educated in using a varying diuretic dose based on their monitoring of symptoms or signs of congestion and their daily weight measurements.
- Thiazide diuretics inhibit the reabsorption of sodium and chloride at the distal portion of nephron. They are less effective in patients with impaired renal function. Although they are less potent than loop diuretics, they may have synergistic action when used with other diuretics.
- Amiloride, triamterene and spironolactone are the potassium-sparing diuretics which act on the distal parts of the nephron, from the late distal tubule to the collecting duct.

  Aldosterone is regarded as the final effector of the renin-angiotensin-aldosterone system that is increased in heart failure. In addition to reabsorption of Na^+, water and secretion of K^+, Aldosterone also is responsible for myocardial fibrosis. Aldosterone has vascular effects including inhibiting the release of nitric oxide.

  Spironolactone, an aldosterone antagonist, is clinically the most commonly used potassium-sparing diuretics that inhibits the aldosterone mediated reabsorption of Na and secretion of K+.
- The RALES trial[26] assessed the effect of spironolactone, used with standard therapy, vs placebo in severe heart failure. Use of spironolactone in severe heart failure was associated with a reduction in mortality and rehospitalisation and improved symptoms of heart failure without increasing safety events. Patients who had severe heart failure with a left ventricular ejection fraction of less than 35% and who were being treated with an angiotensin-converting–enzyme inhibitor were randomly assigned to receive 25 mg of spironolactone daily, and placebo.

  After a mean follow-up period of 24 months, there were 30% reduction in the risk of death and 35% reduction in hospitalisation for worsening heart failure in the spironolactone group than in the placebo group. In addition, patients who received spironolactone had a significant improvement in the symptoms of heart failure.

  Gynaecomastia or breast pain was reported in 10% of men who were treated with spironolactone.

Calcium channel blockers

Non-dihydropyridine calcium channel blockers (e.g. diltiazem, verapamil) are contraindicated in patients with systolic heart failure, owing to their negative inotropic effects. Dihydropyridine calcium channel blockers (amlodipine, felodipine) have not shown survival benefits but may be used to treat co-morbidities (e.g. hypertension) as outcomes are not adverse.

I_f ion channel blocker Ivabradine

- An elevated resting heart rate is an independent predictor of cardiovascular morbidity and mortality, both in the general population and in patients with HF, irrespective of the underlying ejection fraction.[27]
- Ivabradine is a selective inhibitor of the I_f ion channel found in cardiac pacemaker cells of the sinoatrial node. It should be used only for patients in sinus rhythm. Ivabradine lowers the heart rate of patients in sinus rhythm. Its most common side effect is of visual changes (phosphenes); however, it is generally well tolerated. Ivabradine is usually started at 2.5–5.0 mg twice daily and is uptitrated by increasing the dose every 2–4 weeks, aiming for a target dose of 7.5 mg twice daily or the maximum tolerated dose.
- The SHIFT study reported a 10 beats per minute (bpm) reduction in heart rate on top of optimal therapy, which was associated with an 18% relative risk reduction for cardiovascular death and hospital admission for worsening heart failure, in patients with systolic HF, sinus rhythm and a heart rate of 70 bpm or more.[28]
- Ivabradine should be considered in patients with HFrEF associated with an LVEF of ≤35% and with a sinus rate of 70 bpm and above despite receiving maximally tolerated or target doses of an ACE inhibitor (or ARB) and a beta-blocker (unless contraindicated), with or without an MRA. This treatment has been shown to decrease the combined end point of cardiovascular mortality and hospitalisation for HF.[12]

Digoxin

- Digoxin has combined inotropic–bradycardic action. The inotropic effect is due to inhibition of the sodium pump in the myocardial cells. It also slows the sinus node and atrioventricular (AV) node as a result of parasympathetic activation. The extent of the AV nodal inhibitory effect depends on the degree of vagal tone.

- **Haemodynamic effects:** digoxin increases cardiac output, decreases heart rate (it slows AV conduction and prolongs refractory periods by increasing vagal tone) and causes mild vasoconstriction (due to increased cellular calcium). This can include coronary artery vasoconstriction.
- **Pharmacokinetics:** the blood half-life of digoxin is about 36 hours. Digoxin is predominantly excreted by the kidneys unchanged (30% hepatic metabolism). In renal impairment, excretion is decreased and the dose needs to be adjusted. The therapeutic level is 0.5–1.5 ng/mL.[29]
- Digoxin should initially be prescribed at a lower dose (≤0.125 mg daily), and consideration given to checking digoxin levels after 4 weeks. Post-hoc analyses from the Digitalis Investigation Group trial have demonstrated increased mortality associated with higher digoxin levels (≥1.2 ng/mL).[30]
- Although some observational studies have reported increased mortality, digoxin has been shown in randomised controlled trials to have no effect on mortality. Digoxin improved the quality of life and reduced hospitalisation due to heart failure in patients with a left ventricular ejection fraction (LVEF) of ≤45% and in sinus rhythm on top of background therapy, which included diuretics and ACE inhibitors.[31]

Robert was treated with intravenous frusemide and prescribed spironolactone 25 mg daily. His ramipril was uptitrated to 5 mg daily. He was discharged home 5 days later with a follow-up appointment in the community heart failure clinic, where his ramipril was changed to sacubitril/valsartan (Entresto 24/26 mg twice daily) after a 36-hour washout period after his ACE inhibitor ramipril was stopped.

He was advised on:
- *adopting a healthy lifestyle*
- *cessation of alcohol*
- *the importance of adherence to his treatment*
- *monitoring of his symptoms*
- *weighing himself regularly, and*
- *using diuretics in varying doses – an increased dose to be taken if there was worsening dyspnoea or significant weight gain (1–2 kg or more).*

He was also advised to have a regular review by his general practitioner to monitor him for side effects of his medications. Renal function and electrolytes should also be tested regularly when patients are on anti-failure treatment.

He continued to have symptoms of heart failure despite uptitration to the maximum-tolerated guideline-based anti-

failure medications and there was no significant improvement of his left ventricular function.

Questions

1. *What is the role of common antidiabetes medications in presence of heart failure?*
2. *What is Robert's long-term prognosis?*
3. *What is the role of device therapy in improving symptomatic heart failure?*
4. *What are the different device options?*
5. *What is the role of device therapy in improving prognosis?*

Common antidiabetes medications in the presence of heart failure

Metformin is generally safe in heart failure and considered the first-line oral hypoglycaemic agent when diet and lifestyle measures fail to achieve adequate glycaemic control. Metformin is contraindicated in severe renal failure or hepatic impairment owing to the risk of lactic acidosis.

In a systematic review and meta-analysis of published observational studies, the use of **sulfonylureas** was associated with an increased risk of heart failure compared with metformin use.[32] However, indication bias couldn't be ruled out.

Thiazolidinediones (glitazones) are not recommended in a patient with heart failure as they cause sodium and water retention, increasing the risk of HF and hospitalisation, whereas dipeptidylpeptidase-4 (DPP-4) inhibitors have a neutral effect on cardiovascular outcomes. In the SAVOR-TIMI 53 trial, saxagliptin was associated with an increase in risk of hospitalisation for HF, and should not be recommended in patients with type 2 diabetes and a high risk of developing HF.[33-35]

Sodium–glucose co-transporter 2 (SGLT2) inhibitors and **glucagon-like peptide-1 (GLP1) agonists** are antihyperglycaemic agents that have been demonstrated to reduce the risk of cardiovascular events in patients with type 2 diabetes mellitus. GLP1 agonists have a neutral effect on the risk of developing heart failure.

SGLT2 is a sodium–glucose co-transporter in the proximal tubule of the nephron that is responsible for majority of urinary glucose reabsorption. Inhibition of SGLT2 results in glucose lowering as a result of glucosuria. In addition to their effect on blood glucose, SGLT2 inhibitors also cause diuretic and natriuretic effects, weight loss, and lowering of systolic blood pressure.

SGLT2 inhibitors (empagliflozin, canagliflozin or dapagliflozin) are the preferred second-line oral hypoglycaemic agents in a patient with cardiovascular disease and diabetes. In a review and meta-analysis of randomised, placebo-controlled, cardiovascular outcome trials of SGLT2 inhibitors in patients with type 2 diabetes, SGLT2 inhibitors were found to have moderate benefits on major adverse atherosclerotic cardiovascular events.[36] They have robust benefits on reducing hospitalisation for heart failure and progression of renal disease.

In the EMPA-REG OUTCOME trial, empagliflozin significantly reduced the risk of cardiovascular death, non-fatal myocardial infarction or non-fatal stroke by 14% compared with placebo.[37] This reduction was driven mainly by a highly significant 38% reduction in cardiovascular death. In a secondary analysis, empagliflozin was associated with a 35% reduction in hospitalisation for heart failure.

The DAPA-HF trial investigated the role of dapagliflozin in treating patients with an established heart failure with or without diabetes.[38] The trial showed that dapagliflozin reduces death and hospitalisation, and improved health-related quality of life, in patients with HF and reduced ejection fraction.

SGLT2 inhibitors have a diuretic effect and so may increase the effect of loop diuretics and cause intravascular volume contraction. Diuretic dosage may need to be reduced in euvolaemic patients. SGLT2 inhibitors may also increase the risk of mycotic genital infections and euglycaemic ketoacidosis.

Glucagon-like peptide-1 (GLP1) agonists have been shown to decrease cardiovascular events but not heart failure hospitalisation. In a systematic review and meta-analysis, GLP1 receptor agonist treatment showed a significant 10% relative risk reduction in the three-point major adverse cardiovascular event primary outcome (cardiovascular mortality, non-fatal myocardial infarction and non-fatal stroke), a 13% relative risk reduction in cardiovascular mortality and a 12% relative risk reduction in all-cause mortality.[39] No significant effect of GLP1 agonists was identified on fatal and non-fatal myocardial infarction, fatal and non-fatal stroke, or hospital admission for unstable angina or for HF.

PROGNOSIS

- Despite improvement in medical treatment, heart failure remains an important cause of mortality and morbidity, and of recurrent hospital admissions. The AHEAD Main registry, which included 4153 patients hospitalised for acute HF, found the survival rate after day 30 following admission was 79.7% after 1 year and 64.5% after 3 years. Greater age, worse left ventricular dysfunction, co-morbidities and high levels of natriuretic peptides were the most powerful predictors of adverse prognosis and reduced long-term survival.[40]

- In the primary care population, the survival of patients with a diagnosis of HF between 1998 and 2012 was 81.3% (95% confidence interval (CI) 80.9, 81.6), 51.5% (95% CI 51.0, 52.0) and 29.5% (95% CI 28.9, 30.2) at 1, 5 and 10 years respectively – a prognosis similar to that in non-haematological malignancies.[41]

DEVICE THERAPY FOR HEART FAILURE WITH REDUCED SYSTOLIC FUNCTION

- Patients with left ventricular dysfunction are at an increased risk of sudden arrhythmogenic death. The risk of sudden cardiac death (SCD) increases with decreasing left ventricular ejection fraction.[42]
- Patients who have experienced previous sustained ventricular tachyarrhythmias or unexplained syncope are at the greatest risk of SCD.
- In selected patients, device-based therapies are a useful adjunct in systolic heart failure. The most common of these are implantable cardioverter defibrillator (ICD) and cardiac resynchronisation therapy (CRT) pacemakers.
- A single-chamber ICD has a single defibrillator lead implanted in the right ventricle, whereas a dual-chamber ICD has a right atrial pacing lead and a right ventricular defibrillator lead. When an ICD detects ventricular tachyarrhythmia, it initiates therapy by way of antitachycardia pacing or, if required, defibrillation shocks to restore normal rhythm. In addition to antitachycardia therapy and defibrillation shock, ICDs are also capable of back-up pacemaker function for bradyarrhythmias.
- In patients with heart failure, the QRS duration is often considerably prolonged. Intraventricular and interventricular mechanical dyssynchrony may develop as a result of electrical remodelling that, in turn, adversely affects cardiac contractile performance and results in progressive pump failure.
- Cardiac resynchronisation therapy, also commonly known as biventricular pacing, involves simultaneously pacing the left ventricle using an endocardial lead placed via the coronary sinus and a lead in the right ventricle (Fig. 15.5) to restore ventricular synchrony and thus improve left ventricular systolic function.
- These devices have been shown to be useful for the prevention of SCD and progressive pump failure, the two main causes of cardiac mortality in patients with heart failure due to left ventricular dysfunction. Important clinical trials on device therapy in the treatment of HF with systolic dysfunction are shown in Table 15.5.

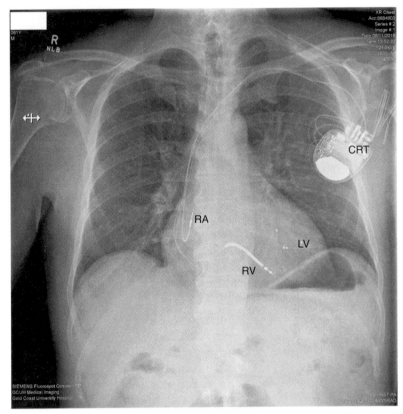

FIG. 15.5 Chest x-ray showing implanted cardiac resynchronisation therapy (CRT) device with endocardial leads in the right atrium (RA) and right ventricle (RV), as well as epicardial coronary sinus lead in the left ventricle (LV).

Implantable Cardioverter Defibrillators

Indications for ICD implantation in patients with heart failure with systolic dysfunction are:

- **Secondary prevention:** following a resuscitated cardiac arrest, an episode of sustained ventricular tachycardia in the presence of haemodynamic compromise or ventricular tachycardia associated with syncope and an LVEF of less than 40%. ICDs have been shown to decrease mortality for these patients.
- **Primary prevention**: an ICD should be considered as primary prevention treatment for patients who have had a myocardial infarction at least 1 month previously and who have an ejection fraction of ≤30%. This has been shown to decrease mortality.[12]
- The benefits of ICD therapy are most significant in patients with ischaemic cardiomyopathy. In the DANISH trial, prophylactic ICD implantation in patients with heart failure and with systolic dysfunc-

tion (left ventricular ejection fraction, ≤35%) due to non-ischaemic cardiomyopathy was not associated with a significantly lower long-term rate of death from any cause than was usual clinical care.[43]

Cardiac Resynchronisation Therapy

Class I indications for CRT in patients with heart failure with reduced systolic function include:

- CRT is recommended in patients with HFrEF associated with sinus rhythm, an LVEF of ≤35% and a QRS duration of 150 ms or more despite optimal medical therapy, to decrease mortality and decrease hospitalisation for heart failure, and to improve symptoms.
- Despite the fact that the benefit of CRT is greater in patients with a broader QRS duration (especially QRS duration ≥150 ms), CRT should be considered in patients with HFrEF associated with sinus rhythm,

TABLE 15.5
Major Clinical Trials on the Use of Device Therapies in Heart Failure

Study	Selection Criteria	Key Findings
IMPLANTABLE CARDIOVERTER DEFIBRILLATOR		
MADIT-II	At least 30 days post myocardial infarction; LV dysfunction; EF <30%	31% reduction of mortality
SCD-HeFT	At least 30 days post myocardial infarction; ischaemic or non-ischaemic NYHA Class II–III; EF <35%	23% reduction of mortality
CARDIAC RESYNCHRONISATION THERAPY		
MADIT-CRT	Mostly NYHA Class II; EF <30%; QRS duration >130 ms	34% reduction of mortality and HF hospitalisation
CARE-HF	Mostly NYHA Class II; EF <35%; QRS duration >120 ms	37% reduction of mortality/cardiovascular hospitalisation
RAFT	Mostly NYHA Class II; EF <30%; QRS duration >120 ms	25% all-cause mortality reduction
IMPLANTABLE CARDIOVERTER DEFIBRILLATOR AND CARDIAC RESYNCHRONISATION THERAPY		
COMPANION trial	NYHA Class III, IV; ischaemic/non-ischaemic cardiomyopathy; QRS duration >120 ms; randomised to medical therapy alone or in combination with CRT or CRT-D	The risk of the combined end point of death or hospitalisation for HF was reduced by 34% in the CRT group and by 40% in the CRT-D group

CRT=cardiac resynchronisation therapy; CRT-D=cardiac resynchronisation therapy with a defibrillator; EF=ejection fraction; HF=heart failure; LV=left ventricle.

(Data from: Moss AJ, Zareba W, Hall WJ, Klein H, Wilber DJ, Cannom DS, et al; Multicenter Automatic Defibrillator Implantation Trial II Investigators. Prophylactic implantation of a defibrillator in patients with myocardial infarction and reduced ejection fraction. N Engl J Med 2002;346:877–83. Bardy GH, Lee KL, Mark DB, Poole JE, Packer DL, Boineau R, et al; Sudden Cardiac Death in Heart Failure Trial (SCD-HeFT) Investigators. Amiodarone or an implantable cardioverter–defibrillator for congestive heart failure. N Engl J Med 2005;352: 225–37; Moss AJ, Hall WJ, Cannom DS, Klein H, Brown MW, Daubert JP, et al; MADIT-CRT Trial Investigators. Cardiac resynchronization therapy for the prevention of heart-failure events. N Engl J Med 2009;361:1329–38; Cleland JG, Daubert JC, Erdmann E, Freemantle N, Gras D, Kappenberger L, et al; Cardiac Resynchronization-Heart Failure (CARE-HF) Study Investigators. The effect of cardiac resynchronization on morbidity and mortality in heart failure. N Engl J Med 2005;352:1539–49; Tang AS, Wells GA, Talajic M, Arnold MO, Sheldon R, Connolly S, et al; Resynchronization–Defibrillation for Ambulatory Heart Failure Trial Investigators. Cardiac-resynchronization therapy for mild-to-moderate heart failure. N Engl J Med 2010;363:2385–95; Bristow MR, Saxon LA, Boehmer J, Krueger S, Kass DA, De Marco T, et al.; Comparison of Medical Therapy, Pacing, and Defibrillation in Heart Failure (COMPANION) Investigators. Cardiac-resynchronization therapy with or without an implantable defibrillator in advanced chronic heart failure. N Engl J Med 2004;350:2140–50.)

an LVEF of ≤35% and a QRS duration of 130–49 ms who remain symptomatic despite optimal medical therapy.

- CRT is contraindicated in patients with QRS duration of less than 130 ms, because it is not effective and may cause harm.[12]

Decisions about pacing, cardiac resynchronisation therapy, defibrillators and the choice of device are complex and generally require specialist review.

Robert was referred to a cardiac electrophysiologist for consideration of a biventricular pacemaker and defibrillator. His ECG following CRT insertion is shown in Fig. 15.6.

Within 4 weeks of the CRT insertion he had an improvement in symptoms and an increased exercise tolerance – about 70% of CRT patients experience significant clinical improvement. A repeat echocardiogram showed resolution of his previous dyssynchrony and an ejection fraction of 40%.

Interrogation of the device showed that he was pacing in both ventricles 100% of the time – biventricular pacing should be present for at least 90% of the time for the treatment to be effective. There had been no detection of any ventricular arrhythmias.

He had regular 6-monthly pacemaker checks and a cardiology review annually.

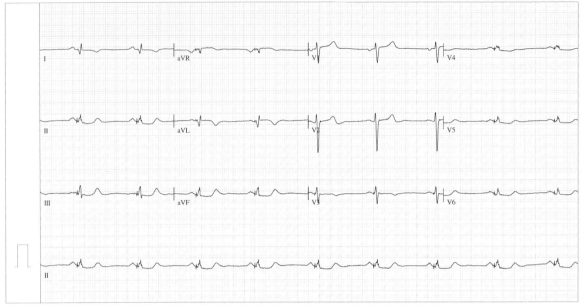

FIG. 15.6 ECG showing sinus rhythm with narrow QRS complex (post-CRT).

He was put in touch with the local heart failure clinic. He was seen there for regular review by a heart failure nurse who was able to advise him about medication changes and his weight, and to provide urgent telephone advice if he felt there had been a significant change in his symptoms. This clinic was also able to help him titrate his drug treatment to the maximum dosages and arrange blood tests of electrolytes and renal function when required.

REFERENCES

1. Yancy CW, Jessup M, Bozkurt B, Butler J, Casey DE Jr, Drazner MH, et al; American College of Cardiology Foundation; American Heart Association Task Force on Practice Guidelines. 2013 ACCF/AHA guideline for the management of heart failure. A report of the American College of Cardiology Foundation/American Heart Association task force on practice guidelines. *J Am Coll Cardiol* 2013;**62**(16): e147–239.
2. Ponikowski P, Voors AA, Anker SD, Bueno H, Cleland JG, Coats AJ, et al; Authors/Task Force Members; Document Reviewers. 2016 ESC Guidelines for the diagnosis and treatment of acute and chronic heart failure: the Task Force for the diagnosis and treatment of acute and chronic heart failure of the European Society of Cardiology (ESC). Developed with the special contribution of the Heart Failure Association (HFA) of the ESC. *Eur J Heart Fail* 2016;**18**:891–975.
3. Chan YK, Tuttle C, Ball J, Teng TK, Ahamed Y, Carrington MJ, et al. Current and projected burden of heart failure in the Australian adult population: a substantive but still ill-defined major health issue. *BMC Health Serv Res* 2016;**16**:501.
4. Bleumink GS, Knetsch AM, Sturkenboom MC, Straus SM, Hofman A, Deckers JW, et al. Quantifying the heart failure epidemic: prevalence, incidence rate, lifetime risk and prognosis of heart failure – The Rotterdam Study. *Eur Heart J* 2004;**25**:1614–19.
5. Gheorghiade M, Sopko G, De Luca L, Velazquez EJ, Parker JD, Binkley PF, et al. Navigating the crossroads of coronary artery disease and heart failure. *Circulation* 2006;**114**:1202–13.
6. Khatibzadeh S, Farzadfar F, Oliver J, Ezzati M, Moran A. Worldwide risk factors for heart failure: a systematic review and pooled analysis. *Int J Cardiol* 2013;**168**(2): 1186–94.
7. Grunig E, Tasman JA, Kücherer H, Franz W, Kübler W, Katus HA. Frequency and phenotypes of familial dilated cardiomyopathy. *J Am Coll Cardiol* 1998;**31**:186–94.
8. Cerqueira MD, Harp GD, Ritchie JL, Stratton JR, Walker RD. Rarity of preclinical alcoholic cardiomyopathy in chronic alcoholics less than 40 years of age. *Am J Cardiol* 1991;**67**:183–7.
9. Bovelli D, Plataniotis G, Roila F. Cardiotoxicity of chemotherapeutic agents and radiotherapy-related heart disease: ESMO Clinical Practice Guidelines. *Ann Oncol* 2010;**21**(Suppl. 5):v277–82.
10. Redfield MM, Jacobsen SJ, Burnett JC, Mahoney DW, Bailey KR, Rodeheffer RJ. Burden of systolic and diastolic

ventricular dysfunction in the community: appreciating the scope of the heart failure epidemic. *JAMA* 2003;**289**(2):194.

11. Fonarow GC, Stough WG, Abraham WT, Albert NM, Gheorghiade M, Greenberg BH, et al; OPTIMIZE-HF Investigators and Hospitals. Characteristics, treatments, and outcomes of patients with preserved systolic function hospitalized for heart failure: a report from the OPTIMIZE-HF Registry. *J Am Coll Cardiol* 2007;**50**:768–77.

12. Atherton JJ, Sindone A, De Pasquale CG, Driscoll A, MacDonald PS, et al; NHFA CSANZ Heart Failure Guidelines Working Group. National Heart Foundation of Australia and Cardiac Society of Australia and New Zealand: guidelines for the prevention, detection, and management of heart failure in Australia 2018. *Heart Lung Circ* 2018;**27**(10): 1123–208.

13. Sato Y, Kita T, Takatsu Y, Kimura T. Biochemical markers of myocyte injury in heart failure. *Heart* 2004;**90**:1110–13.

14. Peacock WF, De Marco T, Fonarow GC, Diercks D, Wynne J, Apple FS, et al; ADHERE Investigators. Cardiac troponin and outcome in acute heart failure. *N Engl J Med* 2008;**358**:2117–26.

15. Davie AP, Francis CM, Love MP, Caruana L, Starkey IR, Shaw TR, et al. Value of the electrocardiogram in identifying heart failure due to left ventricular systolic dysfunction. *BMJ* 1996;**312**:222.

16. Strauss MH, Hall AS. Angiotensin receptor blockers may increase risk of myocardial infarction: unraveling the ARB-MI paradox. *Circulation* 2006;**114**:838–54.

17. Flather MD, Yusuf S, Køber L, Pfeffer M, Hall A, Murray G, et al. Long-term ACE-inhibitor therapy in patients with heart failure or left-ventricular dysfunction: a systematic overview of data from individual patients. ACE-Inhibitor Myocardial Infarction Collaborative Group. *Lancet* 2000; **355**(9215):1575–81.

18. Cohn JN, Tognoni G. A randomized trial of the angiotensin-receptor blocker valsartan in chronic heart failure. *N Engl J Med* 2001;**345**:1667–75.

19. Young JB, Dunlap ME, Pfeffer MA, Probstfield JL, Cohen-Solal A, Dietz R, et al; Candesartan in Heart failure Assessment of Reduction in Mortality and morbidity (CHARM) Investigators and Committees. Mortality and morbidity reduction with candesartan in patients with chronic heart failure and left ventricular systolic dysfunction: results of the CHARM low-left ventricular ejection fraction trials. *Circulation* 2004;**110**:2618–26.

20. Levin ER, Gardner DG, Samson WK. Natriuretic peptides. *N Engl J Med* 1998;**339**:321–8.

21. McMurray JJV, Packer M, Desai AS, Gong J, Lefkowitz MP, Rizkala AR, et al; PARADIGM-HF Investigators and Committees. Angiotensin–neprilysin inhibition versus enalapril in heart failure. *N Engl J Med* 2014;**371**(11):993–1004.

22. Chatterjee K, Parmley WW. The role of vasodilator therapy in heart failure. *Prog Cardiovasc Dis* 1977;**19**:301–25.

23. Cohn JN, Johnson G, Ziesche S, Cobb F, Francis G, Tristani F, et al. A comparison of enalapril with hydralazine – isosorbide dinitrate in the treatment of chronic congestive heart failure. *N Engl J Med* 1991;**325**(5):303–10.

24. Chaggar PS, Malkin CJ, Shaw SM, Williams SG, Channer KS. Neuroendocrine effects on the heart and targets for therapeutic manipulation in heart failure. *Cardiovasc Ther* 2009;**27**:187–93.

25. Cohn JN, Pfeffer MA, Rouleau J, Sharpe N, Swedberg K, Straub M, et al; MOXCON Investigators. Adverse mortality effect of central sympathetic inhibition with sustained-release moxonidine in patients with heart failure (MOXCON). *Eur J Heart Fail* 2003;**5**(5):659–67.

26. Pitt B, Zannad F, Remme WJ, Cody R, Castaigne A, Perez A, et al. The effect of spironolactone on morbidity and mortality in patients with severe heart failure. *N Engl J Med* 1999;**341**:709–17.

27. Kannel WB, Kannel C, Paffenbarger RS Jr, Cupples LA. Heart rate and cardiovascular mortality: the Framingham Study. *Am Heart J* 1987;**113**:1489–94.

28. Swedberg K, Komajda M, Bohm M, Borer JS, Ford I, Dubost-Brama A, et al. Ivabradine and outcomes in chronic heart failure (SHIFT): a randomised placebo-controlled study. *Lancet* 2010;**376**:875–85.

29. Opie LH, Gersh BJ. *Drugs for the heart.* 5th ed. Philadelphia: Elsevier Saunders; 2013.

30. Rathore SS, Curtis JP, Wang Y, Bristow MR, Krumholz HM. Association of serum digoxin concentration and outcomes in patients with heart failure. *JAMA* 2003;**289**:871–8.

31. Digitalis Investigation Group. The effect of digoxin on mortality and morbidity in patients with heart failure. *N Engl J Med* 1997;**336**:525–33.

32. Varas-Lorenzo C, Margulis AV, Pladevall M, Riera-Guardia N, Calingaert B, Hazell L, et al. The risk of heart failure associated with the use of noninsulin blood glucose-lowering drugs: systematic review and meta-analysis of published observational studies. *BMC Cardiovasc Disord* 2014;**14**:129.

33. Hernandez AV, Usmani A, Rajamanickam A, Moheet A. Thiazolidinediones and risk of heart failure in patients with or at high risk of type 2 diabetes mellitus: a meta-analysis and meta-regression analysis of placebo-controlled randomized clinical trials. *Am J Cardiovasc Drugs* 2011;**11**: 115–28.

34. Liu J, Li L, Deng K, Xu C, Busse JW, Vandvik PO, et al. Incretin based treatments and mortality in patients with type 2 diabetes: systematic review and meta-analysis. *BMJ* 2017;**357**:j2499.

35. Scirica BM, Bhatt DL, Braunwald E, Steg PG, Davidson J, Hirshberg B, et al; SAVOR-TIMI 53 Steering Committee and Investigators. Saxagliptin and cardiovascular outcomes in patients with type 2 diabetes mellitus. *N Engl J Med* 2013;**369**:1317–26.

36. Zelniker TA, Wiviott SD, Raz I, Im K, Goodrich EL, Bonaca MP, et al. SGLT2 inhibitors for primary and secondary prevention of cardiovascular and renal outcomes in type 2 diabetes: a systematic review and meta-analysis of cardiovascular outcome trials. *Lancet* 2019;**393**(10166):31–9.

37. Fitchett D, Zinman B, Wanner C, Lachin JM, Hantel S, Salsali A, et al; EMPA-REG OUTCOME® trial investigators. Heart failure outcomes with empagliflozin in patients with type 2 diabetes at high cardiovascular risk: results

of the EMPA-REG OUTCOME® trial. *Eur Heart J* 2016;**37**: 1526–34.

38. McMurray JJV, Solomon SD, Inzucchi SE, Køber L, Kosiborod MN, Martinez FA, et al; DAPA-HF Trial Committees and Investigators. Dapagliflozin in patients with heart failure and reduced ejection fraction. *N Engl J Med* 2019;**381**(21):1995–2008.

39. Bethel MA, Patel RA, Merrill P, Lokhnygina Y, Buse JB, Mentz RJ, et al. Cardiovascular outcomes with glucagon-like peptide-1 receptor agonists in patients with type 2 diabetes: a meta-analysis. *Lancet Diabetes Endocrinol* 2018;**6**: 105–13.

40. Parenica J, Spinar J, Vitovec J, Widimsky P, Linhart A, Fedorco M, et al; AHEAD Main investigators. Long-term survival following acute heart failure: the acute heart failure database main registry (AHEAD main). *Eur J Intern Med* 2013;**24**(2):151–60.

41. Taylor CJ, Ryan R, Nichols L, Gale N, Hobbs FR, Marshall T. Survival following a diagnosis of heart failure in primary care. *Fam Pract* 2017;**34**(2):161–8.

42. Gradman A, Deedwania P, Cody R, Massie B, Packer M, Pitt B, et al. Predictors of total mortality and sudden death in mild to moderate heart failure. Captopril–Digoxin Study Group. *J Am Coll Cardiol* 1989;**14**:564–70.

43. Køber L, Thune JJ, Nielsen JC, Haarbo J, Videbæk L, Korup E, et al; DANISH Investigators. Defibrillator implantation in patients with nonischemic systolic heart failure. *N Engl J Med* 2016;**375**:1221–30.

Syncope

CASE 19 SCENARIO: JESSIE WITH LOSS OF CONSCIOUSNESS

Twenty-three-year-old medical student Jessie presented to the emergency department after brief loss of consciousness. She had collapsed on four occasions in the past 2 years. She has no other medical problem. She had diaphoresis, warmth and nausea, and looked pale before she collapsed.

She was standing for 3 hours in a crowded concert before the event. She recovered quickly; she now feels tired but has no other significant symptoms.

CASE 20 SCENARIO: RHIANNON WITH TRANSIENT LOSS OF CONSCIOUSNESS

Sixty-eight-year-old Rhiannon presented with transient loss of consciousness that occurred while at the dinner table having dinner with her husband.

She had a history of coronary artery disease and previous by-pass surgery 12 years ago. Three weeks ago she

had uncomplicated surgical aortic valve replacement and was discharged home 12 days ago. Her postoperative ECG showed atrial fibrillation. Her medications included aspirin, atorvastatin, perindopril and warfarin.

DEFINITION OF SYNCOPE

- **Syncope** is defined as a transient loss of consciousness (TLOC) due to cerebral hypoperfusion, characterised by rapid onset, short duration and complete spontaneous recovery.[1]
- Syncope is a symptom that presents with an abrupt, transient, complete loss of consciousness, associated with inability to maintain postural tone, with rapid and spontaneous recovery. The presumed mechanism is cerebral hypoperfusion. There should not be clinical features of other non-syncopal causes of loss of consciousness, such as seizure, antecedent head trauma or apparent loss of consciousness (i.e. pseudosyncope).
- **Presyncope (near-syncope)** is the set of symptoms before syncope. These symptoms could include

extreme lightheadedness, visual sensations such as 'tunnel vision' or 'greying out', and variable degrees of altered consciousness without complete loss of consciousness. Presyncope may progress to syncope, or may abort without syncope.[2]

- Syncope is a symptom that can have various causes, ranging from benign to life threatening. Vasovagal syncope is the most common type of syncope.

- Syncope is a common presentation, and population-based studies indicate that approximately 40% of adults have experienced syncope, with women being more likely to report a syncopal event.[3] Reflex (neutrally mediated) syncope is the most common cause of presentation with syncope, followed by cardiac syncope (9%) and syncope due to orthostatic hypotension (9%). Thirty-seven percent of presentations are of undifferentiated syncope.[4]

- Patients with a history of cardiovascular disease, an abnormal electrocardiogram (ECG), a family history of sudden death and those presenting with unexplained syncope should be hospitalised for further diagnostic evaluation. Patients with neurally mediated or orthostatic syncope generally require no additional testing.

CLASSIFICATION OF SYNCOPE BY CAUSE[1]

1. Reflex (neurally mediated)
   - **Vasovagal**
     - Orthostatic – occurs on standing.
     - Emotional – fear, pain, blood, phobia
   - **Situational**
     - Micturition
     - Defecation
     - Cough, sneeze
   - **Carotid sinus syndrome**
   - **Non-classic forms (atypical presentation)**
2. Syncope due to orthostatic hypotension
   - Drug induced (antihypertensives, diuretics)
   - Volume depletion (diarrhoea, vomiting, haemorrhage)
   - Neurogenic orthostatic hypotension
     - Primary autonomic failure (Parkinson disease, dementia with Lewy bodies)
     - Secondary autonomic failure (diabetes, amyloidosis)
   - **Postural orthostatic tachycardia syndrome (POTS):** a clinical syndrome usually characterised by symptoms associated with a heart rate increase >30/min on standing, in the absence of orthostatic hypotension.

3. Cardiac syncope
   - **Bradyarrhythmia** (sinus node dysfunction, high-grade atrioventricular (AV) block)
   - **Tachyarrhythmia** (ventricular or supraventricular)
   - **Inherited arrhythmogenic disorders** (arrhythmogenic right ventricular cardiomyopathy, long QT syndrome, Brugada syndrome)
   - **Structural heart disease** (aortic stenosis, acute myocardial infarction, hypertrophic cardiomyopathy, myxoma, pericardial tamponade, congenital anomalies of the coronary arteries
   - **Cardiopulmonary and great vessel causes** (pulmonary embolus, aortic dissection, pulmonary hypertension)

DIFFERENTIAL DIAGNOSIS OF SYNCOPE

- **Epileptic seizure:** frequently associated with epileptic aura and postictal confusion. Generally, recovery is longer. Patients may have tongue biting and urinary incontinence. They may need to sleep afterwards.
- **Pseudosyncope:** of longer duration; may have a history of psychiatric illness or secondary gain. Examination findings are unremarkable. Episodes often occur when other people are present.
- **Vertebrobasilar transient ischaemic attack (TIA):** may be associated with focal neurological signs.
- **Subarachnoid haemorrhage:** may have accompanying severe headache and neurological signs.
- **Transient loss of consciousness due to head trauma.**
- **Hypoglycaemia:** duration of impaired consciousness is longer. Common in patients with diabetes treated with insulin or oral hypoglycaemic agents. Immediate blood sugar assessment may confirm the diagnosis.
- **Subclavian steal syndrome:** usually due to subclavian artery stenosis proximal to the origin of the vertebral artery. There may be reduced unilateral pulse or blood pressure. Arm exercise induces a syncopal event and other neurological symptoms.

PATHOPHYSIOLOGY OF SYNCOPE

The final common pathway of syncope is reduced systolic blood pressure resulting in cerebral hypoperfusion. A sudden cessation of cerebral blood flow for as little as 6–8 seconds can cause complete loss of consciousness.

Systemic blood pressure is the product of cardiac output and total peripheral resistance; a fall in either can cause syncope.

- **Low cardiac output:** reflex syncope can be caused by reflex bradycardia (cardioinhibitory reflex) due to increased activity of inhibitory receptors and consequent parasympathetic hyperactivity. Low cardiac output syncope also occurs owing to cardiovascular causes including arrhythmias, structural heart disease and pulmonary embolism. Inadequate venous return due to volume depletion, or venous pooling and chronotropic or inotropic incompetence through autonomic failure, may also impair cardiac output and cause syncope.

- **Low peripheral resistance:** decreased reflex activity and withdrawal of sympathetic vascular tone results in vasodilation and decreased blood pressure (vaso-depressive type). Functional or structural impairment of the autonomic nervous system can also cause insufficient vascular tone in response to the upright position and eventual syncope.[1]

ASSESSING A PATIENT WITH SYNCOPE

The initial steps of assessment for patients presenting with syncope are:

- **A detailed history:** in most patients, the cause of syncope can be diagnosed from a detailed history that should include questions about postural, exertional or situational symptoms, palpitations or other cardiac symptoms, a history of previous attacks, eye-witness accounts and even whether a video recording of an episode is available. Bystanders have often been able to record syncopal episodes on their mobile phones. Questions should also be asked about co-morbidities, medication use and past medical conditions, particularly with regards to pre-existing cardiovascular diseases and any family history of sudden cardiac death.
- **Physical examination:** a thorough cardiovascular and neurological examination is the main focus of a physical assessment when investigating a patient with syncope. Examination should include measurement of blood pressure in the supine position and after 3 minutes in the orthostatic position (standing). The presence of a murmur or added heart sound may indicate underlying structural heart disease.

  Carotid sinus massage is indicated in patients >40 years of age with syncope of unknown origin compatible with a reflex mechanism (Class Ib).
- The 12-lead ECG is widely available and inexpensive and can provide information about potential and specific causes of syncope. The ECG may demonstrate bradyarrhythmias, including sinus pauses, high-grade AV block, tachyarrhythmias including atrial fibrillation or flutter with rapid ventricular rate, ventricular

tachycardia, Wolff–Parkinson–White conduction, Brugada syndrome, long QT syndrome, left ventricular hypertrophy, intraventricular conduction defect or the presence of Q waves from previous myocardial infarction (Fig. 16.1). It may also show characteristic ECG features of hypertrophic cardiomyopathy or arrhythmogenic right ventricular cardiomyopathy.

CLINICAL FEATURES THAT CAN SUGGEST A DIAGNOSIS AFTER INITIAL ASSESSMENT
Reflex Syncope

- Vasovagal syncope is typically associated with a prodrome of diaphoresis, warmth and pallor, with fatigue after the event.
- The syncope may occur after prolonged standing, particularly in crowded and hot places. It may occur after exercise (not during exercise).
- There may be a history of recurrent syncope, in particular occurring before the age of 40 years.
- There is often a precipitating factor such as an unpleasant sight or pain.
- Situational syncope is typically triggered by micturition, defecation, cough or sneeze.
- There is generally no history of cardiovascular disease.
- The ECG and cardiovascular examination are usually normal.

Syncope Due to Orthostatic Hypotension

- Syncope occurs during standing and is associated with orthostatic hypotension.
- There may be autonomic neuropathy or parkinsonism.
- There may be a history of vasodilator or diuretic use or a recent increase in dosage.

Cardiac Syncope

- Syncope may occur during exercise (not after exercise) or when supine.
- There are no warning symptoms, or the prodrome is very short.
- There may be the sudden onset of palpitations followed by syncope.
- There may be a family history of sudden cardiac death.
- The patient may be known to have a history of left ventricular dysfunction, structural heart disease or previous myocardial infarction.
- The cardiovascular examination is often abnormal (murmur or other signs of structural heart disease, unexplained bradycardia or tachycardia, or hypoxia).
- The ECG is often abnormal.

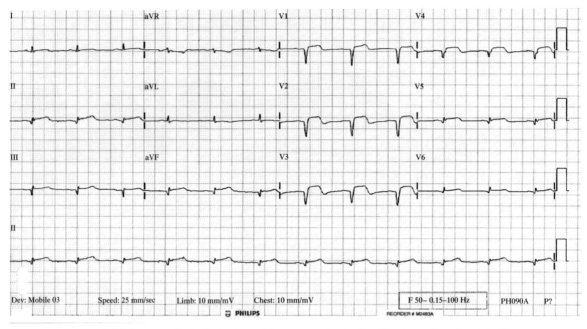

FIG. 16.1 ECG from a patient who had a sudden syncopal episode without warning, showing old anterior and inferior infarcts. It raises the possibility of a ventricular arrhythmia as the cause of the episode.

INVESTIGATING A PATIENT WITH SYNCOPE

The history, physical examination and electrocardiography are the core of the initial syncope work-up, with a combined diagnostic yield of 50%.[5]

Active Standing

This test is used to diagnose orthostatic intolerance. The heart rate and blood pressure (BP) are recorded while the patient is supine and during 3 minutes of standing. This should be done at the initial syncope evaluation. An abnormal BP fall is defined as a progressive and sustained fall in systolic BP from baseline value >20 mmHg or diastolic BP >10 mmHg, or a decrease in systolic BP to <90 mmHg.

Ambulatory BP Monitoring

There is evidence that 24-hour ambulatory BP monitoring is useful in diagnosing orthostatic hypotension due to autonomic failure where there is often associated nocturnal hypertension (non-dipping pattern).[6]

Electrocardiographic Monitoring

In-hospital monitoring is indicated when an arrhythmia-associated syncope is suspected.

- The Holter monitor, a portable, battery-operated device that records continuously for 24–72 hours (some of the newer devices record longer times) has a low yield in identifying the cause of syncope. It can be particularly helpful if the symptoms are frequent. A patient-activated event diary is useful to confirm arrhythmic cause of syncope when a correlation between syncope and arrhythmias is detected.

- An external loop recorder is a device that continuously records and stores data, and can be patient activated or auto triggered. External loop recording is helpful when there is a pattern of an intersymptom interval of a few weeks.

- The internal loop recorder, a subcutaneously implanted device with a battery life of 2–3 years, is useful in patients with recurrent syncope (Fig. 16.2) after a non-diagnostic initial workup when the events are infrequent and an arrhythmia (bradyarrhythmia or tachyarrhythmia) is suspected to be the cause, but the indications for primary prevention with an implantable cardioverter defibrillator (ICD) or pacemaker are not met. Arrhythmic syncope is diagnosed when a correlation between syncope and an arrhythmia is detected.

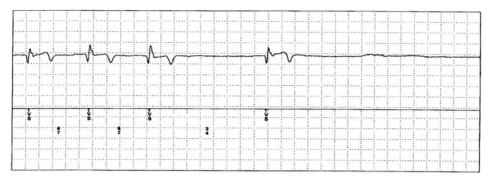

FIG. 16.2 Internal loop recorder trace in a patient with recurrent syncope.

Exercise Stress Test (EST)

The EST is frequently used as a screening tool for the detection and risk stratification of coronary artery disease. Exercise testing may also be helpful in unexplained syncope, where the episodes occur during or shortly after exercise. Exercise testing provides information on BP and pulse rate response to exercise. Patients may develop high-grade AV block during exercise, or other exercise-induced arrhythmias. Reflex syncope is confirmed when syncope is reproduced immediately after exercise in the presence of severe hypotension.

Head-Up Tilt Table Test (HUTT)

The HUTT is used in patients with suspected reflex syncope, orthostatic hypotension or POTS and also in psychogenic pseudosyncope. It involves simultaneous monitoring of the cardiac rhythm and blood pressure while the patient is placed at 60–70 degrees for, typically, more than 30 minutes. If no event is reproduced and vital signs remain normal, testing is repeated with a pharmacological challenge (sublingual glyceryl trinitrate). The test is considered positive if the symptoms are replicated when the patient develops hypotension and bradycardia. Unfortunately, a negative HUTT does not exclude a diagnosis of reflex syncope.

Echocardiography and Other Cardiac Imaging Modality

The choice of cardiac imaging modality depends on the disease being investigated, individual patient characteristics and the accessibility of tests locally. Echocardiography is a widely available test indicated for the diagnosis and risk stratification of suspected structural heart disease (e.g. severe aortic stenosis, hypertrophic cardiomyopathy, obstructive cardiac tumours or thrombi, pericardial tamponade or aortic dissection).[1] Echocardiography is most useful in patients with unexplained syncope and a positive cardiac history or abnormal ECG.[7]

- Exercise stress echocardiogram is useful to detect exercise-induced left ventricular outflow obstruction in patients with hypertrophic cardiomyopathy and a history of exertional syncope.
- Computed tomography (CT) and cardiac magnetic resonance imaging (MRI) should be considered in selected patients presenting with syncope of suspected cardiac structural origin when echocardiography is not diagnostic. CT coronary angiography is useful to investigate a suspected anomalous coronary artery in a patient with syncope. This is a cause of exertional syncope and sudden cardiac death, classically in young athletes.
- MRI is useful in identifying myocardial fibrosis and inflammation. Cardiac MRI is particularly useful in suspected myocarditis, arrhythmogenic right ventricular cardiomyopathy or sarcoidosis.

Electrophysiological (EP) Study

The strong indication (class I) for the use of an implantable cardiac defibrillator for primary prevention of sudden cardiac death in patients with ischaemic cardiomyopathy and ejection fractions <35% has resulted in a diminished role of the EP study in the evaluation of ventricular arrhythmias.[2]

In patients with syncope and previous myocardial infarction or other scar-related conditions, an EP study is recommended when symptoms remain unexplained after non-invasive tests.[1]

The EP study remains useful in selected patients with asymptomatic sinus bradycardia, suspected sinus arrest causing syncope, bifascicular block and suspected tachyarrhythmias.[1]

In patients with unexplained syncope and bifascicular block, an EP study is useful in identifying patients with intermittent high-degree AV block or impending high-grade AV block. The H–V interval can be used to evaluate the conduction in the remaining fibres. A relatively short H–V interval (<70 ms) implies normal conduction through the remaining fibres, whereas a prolonged H–V interval (>70 ms) implies impaired conduction through the remaining fibres and is an indication for a pacemaker to be fitted.

An EP study is not helpful in a patient with syncope who has a normal ECG and normal cardiac structure and function, unless an arrhythmic aetiology is suspected.[2]

MANAGEMENT OF VASOVAGAL SYNCOPE

Most of the patients with initial assessment suggesting reflex syncope or syncope due to orthostatic hypotension can be discharged from the ED and investigated in the community. On the other hand, features suggesting a cardiac cause of syncope mean prompt evaluation is necessary.[1]

Non-Pharmacological Treatment

Initial therapy of vasovagal syncope is non-pharmacological. Patient should identify and avoid the triggers. If possible they should lie down if they recognise the onset of prodromal symptoms. Physical counter-manoeuvres like leg crossing, limb and abdominal contraction and squatting, which improve venous return, can be helpful.[8] Fluid intake should be increased by up to 2–2.5 L per day and, unless the patient has a history of heart failure or hypertension, salt intake should also be increased. A review of medication (particularly of antihypertensive drugs, diuretics, psychotropic drugs and alpha-blockers used for symptoms of prostatic hypertrophy) for possible side effects should be undertaken in older patients. A 24-hour ambulatory blood pressure could help to identify pseudohypertension and optimise antihypertensive drug dosage. Compression stockings may be helpful in some patients but are often associated with poor adherence. Patients also need to be reassured about the benign nature of the condition. Patients with vasovagal syncope have a long-term risk of death similar to that of risk-matched patients without syncope.[4]

Pharmacological Treatment
Alpha-agonist (midodrine)
- The peripherally active alpha-agonist midodrine can be used to increase peripheral vascular tone. A meta-analysis of randomised controlled trials showed a significant reduction in recurrence of syncope with midodrine treatment.[9]

Beta-blockers
- The use of beta-blockers has been suggested for patients with vasovagal syncope on the presumption that they reduce ventricular mechanoreceptor activation, but, unfortunately, the results from trials on the use of beta-blockers in the prevention of vasovagal syncope have been disappointing. In the Prevention of Syncope Trial (POST) there was a suggestion that beta-blockers are effective in suppressing vasovagal syncope in patients older than 42 years, and a subsequent meta-analysis supports this.[10,11]
- Current ACC/AHA/HRS syncope guidelines suggest beta-blocker use is reasonable in patients 42 years of age or older with recurrent vasovagal syncope (class IIb indication).[2] However, ESC guidelines for the diagnosis and management of syncope recommend 'There is sufficient evidence from multiple trials that beta-blockers are not appropriate in reducing syncopal recurrences.'[1]

Fludrocortisone
- Fludrocortisone has been demonstrated to reduce recurrences of vasovagal syncope in young patients due to frequent vasovagal syncope in the POST 2 trial (Prevention of Syncope Trial 2), a randomised, double-blind, placebo-controlled study of fludrocortisone in the prevention of vasovagal syncope.[12] Fludrocortisone has mineralocorticoid properties and causes sodium and water retention, potassium excretion and increased blood volume. The serum potassium level should be monitored because of potential drug-induced hypokalaemia. Fludrocortisone should not be used in patients with heart failure or hypertension.

Selective serotonin reuptake inhibitor (SSRI)
- In patients with recurrent vasovagal syncope, a SSRI might be considered. Unfortunately, small randomised controlled trials on selective serotonin inhibitors in the treatment of vasovagal syncope have showed conflicting results.[13,14]

Pacemakers in Vasovagal Syncope
Vasovagal syncope is often associated with a cardioinhibitory response (bradycardia and asystole) and, therefore, pacemakers have been proposed as a potential treatment in selected patients. There is still debate, however, regarding which patients will benefit from a pacemaker insertion. Previous randomised controlled trials did not show any statistically significant benefit from pacing.[15,16]

However, in the randomised double-blind third International Study on Syncope of Uncertain Etiology (ISSUE)-3 trial,[17] patients who had syncope with >3-second period of asystole or >6-second period of asystole without syncope were randomly assigned to receive either dual chamber pacing with rate drop response or sensing only. The trial showed a 32% absolute and a 57% relative reduction in recurrence of syncope in the pacing group.

Based on this trial, in selected patients more than 40 years of age, a dual chamber pacemaker should be considered to reduce recurrence of syncope when the correlation between symptoms and ECG is established.[1] Similarly, despite lack of large randomised controlled trials, there is sufficient evidence that a dual chamber pacemaker should be considered to reduce syncope recurrence in patients affected by dominant cardioinhibitory carotid sinus syndrome.[1]

TREATMENT OF CARDIAC SYNCOPE

Treatment of cardiac syncope depends on the underlying cause. Syncope due to severe aortic stenosis or hypertrophic obstructive cardiomyopathy is treated by surgical or percutaneous aortic valve replacement and septal myomectomy or alcohol septal ablation respectively. Hypertrophic cardiomyopathy patients may develop syncope as a result of ventricular arrhythmias, and for these an ICD may be indicated. Similarly, depending on the underlying cause, treatment of arrhythmogenic cardiac syncope could be antiarrhythmic medications, a pacemaker insertion or a defibrillator.

Jessie's physical examination was unremarkable except the supine blood pressure 98/60 mmHg without any postural drop. Her pulse rate was 70/minute with no significant change on standing. Her ECG showed sinus rhythm. She had no ECG evidence of left ventricular hypertrophy or abnormal Q waves. Her P–R interval and Q–Tc interval were normal. She did not have a delta wave or a Brugada-type ECG. She was diagnosed with vasovagal syncope, reassured and discharged home with advice on avoidance of precipitants and on non-pharmacological precautions.

Due to her previous ischaemic heart disease and by-pass surgery, recent aortic valve replacement and nature of unprovoked syncope while sitting, Rhiannon likely had cardiac syncope. Calcific aortic stenosis is associated with cardiac conduction abnormalities as a result of calcification extending from the annulus of the aortic valve into the conducting system (Lev's syndrome). Her ECG (Fig. 16.3) showed dissociation of P waves and QRS complexes, suggesting complete heart block. She had a dual chamber pacemaker inserted as an inpatient and was discharged home the next day.

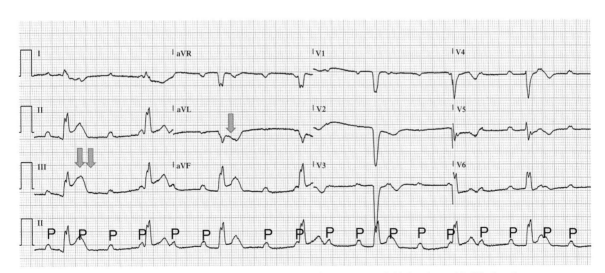

FIG. 16.3 complete heart block complicating acute inferior myocardial infarction, with ST elevation (double arrow) in LII, LIII and aVF with reciprocal ST depression (single arrow) in LI and aVL. There is no relationship between the P waves and QRS complexes, suggesting complete heart block.

REFERENCES

1. Brignole M, Moya A, de Lange FJ, Deharo JC, Elliott PM, Fanciulli A, et al; ESC Scientific Document Group. 2018 ESC guidelines for the diagnosis and management of syncope. *Eur Heart J* 2018;**39**:1883–948.
2. Shen WK, Sheldon RS, Benditt DG, Cohen MI, Forman DE, Goldberger ZD, et al. 2017 ACC/AHA/HRS Syncope Guideline: executive summary. *Circulation* 2017;**136**:e60–122.
3. Parry SW, Tan MP. An approach to the evaluation and management of syncope in adults. *BMJ* 2010;**340**:c880.
4. Soteriades ES, Evans JC, Larson MG, Chen MH, Chen L, Benjamin EJ, et al. Incidence and prognosis of syncope. *N Engl J Med* 2002;**347**:878–85.
5. Linzer M, Yang EH, Estes NA III, Wang P, Vorperian VR, Kapoor WN. Diagnosing syncope. Part 1: value of history, physical examination, and electrocardiography. Clinical Efficacy Assessment Project of the American College of Physicians. *Ann Intern Med* 1997;**126**(12):989–96.
6. Voichanski S, Grossman C, Leibowitz A, Peleg E, Koren-Morag N, Sharabi Y, et al. Orthostatic hypotension is associated with nocturnal change in systolic blood pressure. *Am J Hypertens* 2012;**25**:159–64.
7. Sarasin FP, Junod AF, Carballo D, Slama S, Unger PF, Louis-Simonet M. Role of echocardiography in the evaluation of syncope: a prospective study. *Heart* 2002;**88**(4):363–7.
8. Van Dijk N, Quartieri F, Blanc JJ, Garcia-Civera R, Brignole M, Moya A, et al; PC-Trial Investigators. Effectiveness of physical counterpressure maneuvers in preventing vasovagal syncope: the Physical Counterpressure Manoeuvres Trial (PC-Trial). *J Am Coll Cardiol* 2006;**48**:1652–7.
9. Vyas A, Swaminathan PD, Zimmerman MB, Olshansky B. Are treatments for vasovagal syncope effective? A meta-analysis. *Int J Cardiol* 2013;**167**:1906–11.
10. Sheldon R, Connolly S, Rose S, Klingenheben T, Krahn A, Morillo C, et al. Prevention of Syncope Trial (POST): a randomized, placebo-controlled study of metoprolol in the prevention of vasovagal syncope. *Circulation* 2006;**113**:1164–70.
11. Sheldon RS, Morillo CA, Klingenheben T, Krahn AD, Sheldon A, Rose MS. Age-dependent effect of beta-blockers in preventing vasovagal syncope. *Circ Arrhythm Electrophysiol* 2012;**5**:920–6.
12. Sheldon R, Raj SR, Rose MS, Morillo CA, Krahn AD, Medina E, et al. Fludrocortisone for the prevention of vasovagal syncope: a randomized, placebo-controlled trial. *J Am Coll Cardiol* 2016;**68**:1–9.
13. Di Girolamo E, Di Iorio C, Sabatini P, Morillo CA, Krahn AD, Medina E, et al; POST 2 Investigators. Effects of paroxetine hydrochloride, a selective serotonin reuptake inhibitor, on refractory vasovagal syncope: a randomized, double-blind, placebo-controlled study. *J Am Coll Cardiol* 1999;**33**:1227–30.
14. Takata TS, Wasmund SL, Smith ML, Li JM, Joglar JA, Banks K, et al. Serotonin reuptake inhibitor does not prevent the vasovagal reaction associated with carotid sinus massage and/or lower body negative pressure in healthy volunteers. *Circulation* 2002;**106**:1500–4.
15. Connolly SJ, Sheldon R, Thorpe KE, Roberts RS, Ellenbogen KA, Wilkoff BL, et al. VPS II Investigators. Pacemaker therapy for prevention of syncope in patients with recurrent severe vasovagal syncope: second Vasovagal Pacemaker Study (VPS II): a randomized trial. *JAMA* 2003;**289**:2224–9.
16. Raviele A, Giada F, Menozzi C, Speca G, Orazi S, Gasparini G, et al; Vasovagal Syncope and Pacing Trial Investigators. A randomized, double-blind, placebo-controlled study of permanent cardiac pacing for the treatment of recurrent tilt-induced vasovagal syncope. The vasovagal syncope and pacing trial (SYNPACE). *Eur Heart J* 2004;**25**:1741–8.
17. Brignole M, Menozzi C, Moya A, Andresen D, Blanc JJ, Krahn AD, et al; International Study on Syncope of Uncertain Etiology 3 (ISSUE-3) Investigators. Pacemaker therapy in patients with neurally mediated syncope and documented asystole: third International Study on Syncope of Uncertain Etiology (ISSUE-3): a randomized trial. *Circulation* 2012;**125**:2566–71.

CHAPTER 17

Coronavirus Disease 2019

KEY POINTS

- Coronavirus disease 2019 (COVID-19) is caused by severe acute respiratory syndrome coronavirus 2 (SARS-CoV-2) with a mean incubation period of 4 days.
- Fever is the most common symptom, occurring in up to 98.6% of the patients during the course of the illness.
- Lymphocytopenia is common and the majority of patients have bilateral ground-glass opacity on a chest computed tomography (CT) scan.
- The majority of the infections are classified as mild and just 5% of patients may develop serious complications, including respiratory failure, myocarditis, shock and/or multiorgan dysfunction. The overall mortality for confirmed cases is 1.38%, which rises sharply with age.
- Cardiovascular complications, including myocardial injury, myocarditis and both type 1 myocardial infarction (MI), due to a plaque rupture, and type 2 MI, due to myocardial supply/demand mismatch, have been described.
- Although COVID-19 virus binds to the angiotensin-converting enzyme 2 (ACE2) receptor to gain entry into cells, medications including the ACE inhibitors and angiotensin receptor blockers (ARBs) do not increase the risk of contracting COVID-19.

CASE 21 SCENARIO: PETER WITH DYSPNOEA, DRY COUGH AND FEVER

76-year-old Peter was referred to the hospital's emergency department with increasing dyspnoea, a dry cough and fever. He also has myalgia, nausea, abdominal discomfort and diarrhoea. His chest x-ray shows bilateral lower-zone infiltrate. He had returned from a cruise 5 days previously.

The coronavirus disease 2019 (COVID-19) is caused by severe acute respiratory syndrome coronavirus 2 (SARS-CoV-2), with the case being reported in December 2019. The World Health Organization declared the COVID-19 outbreak a pandemic on 11 March 2020.

- The mean incubation period of the COVID-19 is 4 days (interquartile range: 2–7).[1] A majority of the patients develop symptoms within 11.5 days after exposure.[2] Almost all cases develop symptoms within 14 days after exposure to the virus.
- Although the majority of the earlier cases were linked to the Huanan Seafood Wholesale Market and the patients could have been infected through zoonotic or environmental exposures, it is now established that the virus has the ability of a robust human-to-human transmission, primarily via close contact and through

respiratory droplets. There is also report of possible faecal–oral transmission.[3]

SYMPTOMS

The clinical presentation and the symptom severity vary, ranging from mild non-specific flu-like symptoms to a severe viral pneumonia leading to potential fatal acute respiratory distress syndrome (ARDS), shock and death.[1,4]

- Fever is the most common symptom at onset of illness in all studies, occurring in 43.8% of patients on hospital admission and 88.7%–98.6% during hospitalisation. Some patients may have a very-low-grade fever.
- Dry cough is seen in 59.4%–68.7%.
- Dyspnoea is present in 31.2% of patients. The median durations from first symptoms to dyspnoea is 5 days, and to intensive care unit (ICU) admission it is 10 days.
- Other symptoms include myalgia, fatigue, sore throat, anorexia, nausea, vomiting, diarrhoea and other gastrointestinal symptoms.
- Those patients who require an ICU admission are generally older and are more likely to have underlying

co-morbidities, including hypertension, diabetes, cardiovascular disease and cerebrovascular diseases.

INVESTIGATIONS

- Lymphocytopenia is present in 83.2% of patients on admission. Thrombocytopenia, prolonged prothrombin time, elevated lactate dehydrogenase (LD), elevated C-reactive protein (CRP) and other markers of inflammation, elevated liver enzymes (alanine aminotransferase and aspartate aminotransferase) and elevated troponin are also common findings. In addition to decreased lymphocyte count, patients who die from the illness also frequently have increased neutrophil, D-dimer, blood urea and creatinine levels.
- Chest radiographs may be normal in the early or mild stages of the disease. Of the patients requiring hospitalisation due to COVID-19, 80% may have radiographic abnormalities at some time during hospitalisation. Chest radiographs typically reveal bilateral, peripheral, lower-zone opacities or, less commonly, ground-glass opacity.[5]
- On admission, ground-glass opacity is the most common radiological finding on a chest computed tomography (CT scan). Bilateral patchy infiltrate (Fig. 17.1) is also common.[6] The initial chest CT scan shows abnormalities in at least 85% of patients.

COURSE AND COMPLICATIONS

- The exact clinical course, severity and complications of COVID-19 are not yet completely determined. Wu and colleagues reported from China that 81% of

infections were classified as mild, 14% as severe and only 5% as critical, which was defined as having respiratory failure, septic shock and/or multiorgan dysfunction.[7]
- The comprehensive study of COVID-19 deaths and hospitalisations has revealed an overall death rate for confirmed cases of 1.38%, which rose sharply with age (0.32% in those aged <60 years vs 6.4% in those aged >60 and 7.8% in those over 80 years of age).[8]

CARDIOVASCULAR CONDITIONS AND COVID-19 INFECTION

The cardiovascular manifestations directly related to COVID-19 include myocardial injury, severe myocarditis/myopericarditis with or without pericardial effusion, acute coronary syndrome, cardiomyopathy, congestive heart failure (CHF), cardiogenic shock, supraventricular and ventricular arrhythmias and thromboembolic disease including deep vein thrombosis (DVT) and pulmonary embolism. Those with underlying cardiovascular disease (CVD) have a higher risk of contracting COVID-19 and a worse prognosis.

Elevated Biomarkers: Troponin and Natriuretic Peptides

- Mild elevation of troponin in hospitalised patients with COVID-19 is common and frequently correlates with disease severity, and is a marker for cardiac involvement. Cardiac biomarker studies suggest a high prevalence of cardiac injury in hospitalised patients. In a study of 416 hospitalised patients, 19.7% had

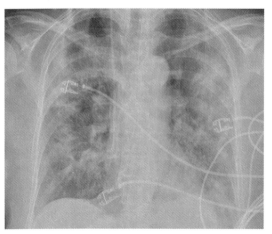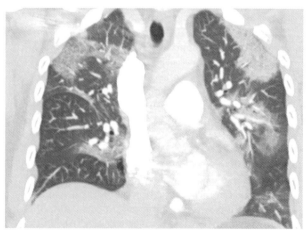

FIG. 17.1 Chest X-Ray (left) in a COVID-19 patient, showing bilateral patchy infiltrate. On the right the corresponding computed tomography (CT scan)showing typical ground-glass opacity (coronal sections). (Courtesy Dr Hasan Shohag, GCUH.)

evidence of myocardial injury manifested by elevation of high-sensitivity troponin I (TnI) levels.[9] Patients with cardiac injury had a higher mortality.

- The cause of troponin elevation in serious infection is multifactorial. It has been suggested that inflammatory cytokines released from neutrophils, particularly tumour necrosis factor alpha (TNF-α) and interleukin 6 (IL-6), are responsible for direct myocardial depression and increased cell membrane permeability to troponin molecules in sepsis.[10]
- Decreased myocardial perfusion due to hypotension, increased oxygen consumption due to tachycardia, release of noradrenaline and adrenaline with subsequent vasoconstriction and increased coagulation of the capillary bed have all been proposed as playing a significant part in myocyte damage and subsequent troponin release.[11]
- A recent statement by the American College of Cardiology (ACC) suggests that a rise and/or fall of highly sensitive troponin is not sufficient to secure the diagnosis of acute myocardial infarction (MI), which should be based on clinical judgment, symptoms/signs and ECG changes. Investigations such as echocardiography or coronary angiography for COVID-19 patients with elevated biomarkers should be restricted to those in whom these procedures are expected to influence the clinical decision making.
- Natriuretic peptides (B-type natriuretic peptide (BNP) or *N*-terminal-prohormone B-type natriuretic peptide (NT-proBNP)) are biomarkers of myocardial stress and are frequently elevated among patients with severe respiratory illnesses, typically in the absence of elevated filling pressures or clinical heart failure. Similar to troponin, elevation of BNP or NT-proBNP is associated with an unfavourable course among patients with ARDS.[12]

Acute Coronary Syndrome

- Both type 1 MI (due to a plaque rupture) and type 2 MI (due to myocardial supply/demand mismatch because of tachycardia, hypoxia from ARDS and potential microthrombi triggered by the COVID-19 infection) are possible.
- Case reports have been published that describe patients with COVID-19 presenting with ECG findings suggesting ST elevation MI (STEMI) or with non–ST elevation MI (NSTEMI) without angiographic evidence of obstructive coronary artery disease.[13]
- According to recently released consensus guidelines from the Cardiac Society of Australia and New Zealand, thrombolytic therapy may be considered (preferred) in patients with suspected COVID-19 and STEMI.

- Though treating a patient with NSTEMI using a strategy of early invasive coronary angiography may reduce recurrent MI, angina and hospitalisation, there is no evidence that early intervention reduces death or non-fatal MI. There is also no evidence to support the use of early invasive coronary angiography amongst patient with type 2 MI. Patients need to be assessed on a case-by-case basis and a low-risk patient should be considered for medical treatment. During the pandemic, strict infection control measures to limit infection spread within the hospital and among healthcare workers should be an important consideration.
- ECG changes, including both tachyarrhythmia and bradyarrhythmia, have frequently been described in COVID-19-infected patients. Among hospitalised patients with COVID-19, 26.1% patients required ICU admission because of complications, including arrhythmias in 44% of the patients.[4]
- No data exist to suggest a benefit from antiplatelet or anticoagulant therapy for those with acute myocardial injury due to type 2 MI.[12]

Cardiomyopathy and Heart Failure

- Among the severely and critically ill hospitalised patients with COVID-19, cardiomyopathy, associated heart failure and cardiogenic shock have been reported. These patients have an extremely high mortality rate and usually require cardiopulmonary support. There is report of infiltration of the myocardium by mononuclear inflammatory cells. The exact mechanism of cardiac involvement in COVID-19 remains unclear. One potential mechanism is direct myocardial involvement mediated via ACE2. Given that increased interleukin levels are frequently observed in such patients, it is also possible that the mechanisms of COVID-19-related cardiac involvement include a cytokine storm due to hyperinflammation.[14]
- Heart failure was observed in 23.0% of patients with COVID-19 presentations.[15]
- In a case report of 138 hospitalised patients with COVID-19, 16.7% developed arrhythmias, 7.2% developed myocardial injury (elevated troponin I, new ECG changes or echocardiographic abnormalities) and 8.7% developed shock requiring vasopressors.[4]

Renin-active Agents in COVID-19 Infection

- Hypertension and coronary heart disease (CAD) are common amongst COVID-19 sufferers, indicating poorer clinical prognosis. Both hypertension and CAD are often treated with angiotensin-converting enzyme (ACE) inhibitors or angiotensin receptor blockers (ARBs).

- Infection with COVID-19 virus is caused by binding of a spike protein on the viral surface to the ACE2 receptor. Studies involving rodent models have shown that treatment with ACE inhibitors (ACEIs) or ARBs may lead to an increase in ACE2.
- There is concern that renin–angiotensin–aldosterone system antagonists such as ACEIs and ARBs could increase a patient's susceptibility to the virus by upregulating ACE2.[16]
- The position statement of the European Society of Cardiology (ESC) Council on Hypertension on an ACEI and ARBs 'strongly recommend that physicians and patients should continue treatment with their usual anti-hypertensive therapy because there is no clinical or scientific evidence to suggest that treatment with ACEI or ARBs should be discontinued because of the COVID-19 infection'.[17] The American College of Cardiology and the American Heart Association have also made similar recommendation.

TREATMENT

Treatment of serious COVID-19 infection is mainly supportive. Using standard public health and personal hygiene strategies for preventing the spread of the disease remains the priority.

A number of clinical trials are currently ongoing to ascertain the efficacy of different antiviral, antimalarial/immunomodulator drugs, IL-6 inhibitors, high-dose corticosteroids and convalescent plasma. Patients should be encouraged to enrol to these clinical trials when possible.

Peter received supportive care in the hospital. In addition, he was enrolled onto a clinical trial. He was discharged on day 5, when he was placed on home isolation. He was regularly reviewed by virtual clinic.

REFERENCES

1. Guan VW, Ni Z, Hu Y, Liang W, Ou C, He J, et al; for the China Medical Treatment Expert Group for Covid-19. Clinical characteristics of coronavirus disease 2019 in China. *N Engl J Med* 2020; Online ahead of print.
2. Lauer SA, Grantz KH, Bi Q, Jones FK, Zheng Q, Meredith HR, et al. The incubation period of coronavirus disease 2019 (COVID-19) from publicly reported confirmed cases: estimation and application. *Ann Intern Med* 2020; M20-0504, Online ahead of print.
3. Li Q, Guan X, Wu P, Wang X, Zhou L, Tong Y, et al. Early transmission dynamics in Wuhan, China, of novel coronavirus–infected pneumonia. *N Engl J Med* 2020; **382**(13):1199–207.
4. Wang D, Hu B, Hu C, Zhu F, Liu X, Zhang J, et al. Clinical characteristics of 138 hospitalized patients with 2019 novel corona virus–infected pneumonia in Wuhan, China. *JAMA* 2020;**323**(11):1061–9.
5. Wong HYF, Lam HYS, Fong AH, Leung ST, Chin TW, Lo CSY, et al. Frequency and distribution of chest radiographic findings in COVID-19 positive patients. *Radiology* 2019; Online ahead of print.
6. Hosseiny M, Kooraki S, Gholamrezanezhad A, Reddy S, Myers L. Radiology perspective of coronavirus disease 2019 (COVID-19): lessons from severe acute respiratory syndrome and Middle East Respiratory Syndrome. *AJR Am J Roentgenol* 2020;1–5. Online ahead of print.
7. Wu Z, McGoogan JM. Characteristics of and important lessons from the coronavirus disease 2019 (COVID-19) outbreak in China: summary of a report of 72 314 cases from the Chinese Center for Disease Control and Prevention. *JAMA* 2020; Online ahead of print.
8. Verity R, Okell LC, Whittaker C, Imai N. Estimates of the severity of coronavirus disease 2019: a model-based analysis. *Lancet Infect Dis* 2020; Online ahead of print.
9. Shi S, Qin M, Shen B, Cai Y, Liu T, Yang F, et al. Association of cardiac injury with mortality in hospitalized patients with COVID-19 in Wuhan, China. *JAMA Cardiol* 2020; Online ahead of print.
10. Zanotti-Cavazzoni SL, Hollenberg SM. Cardiac dysfunction in severe sepsis and septic shock. *Curr Opin Crit Care* 2009;**15**:392–7.
11. Kalla C, Raveh D, Algur N, Rudensky B, Yinnon AM, Balkin J. Incidence and significance of a positive troponin test in bacteremic patients without acute coronary syndrome. *Am J Med* 2008;**121**:909–15.
12. Januzzi JL Jr. Troponin and BNP use in COVID-19. *Am Coll Cardiol* 2020; https://www.acc.org/latest-in-cardiology/articles/2020/03/18/15/25/troponin-and-bnp-use-in-covid19.
13. Hu H, Ma F, Wei X, Fang Y. Coronavirus fulminant myocarditis treated with glucocorticoid and human immunoglobulin. *Eur Heart J* 2020; Online ahead of print.
14. Mehta P, McAuley DF, Brown M, Sanchez E, Tattersall RS, Manson JJ, et al; HLH Across Speciality Collaboration, UK. COVID-19: consider cytokine storm syndromes and immunosuppression. *Lancet* 2020;**395**(10229):1033–4.
15. Zhou F, Yu T, Du R, et al. Clinical course and risk factors for mortality of adult inpatients with COVID-19 in Wuhan, China: a retrospective cohort study. *Lancet* 2020;**395**(10229):1054–62.
16. Ferrario CM, Jessup J, Chappell MC, Averill DB, Brosnihan KB, Tallant EA, et al. Effect of angiotensin-converting enzyme inhibition and angiotensin II receptor blockers on cardiac angiotensin-converting enzyme 2. *Circulation* 2005;**111**:2605–10.
17. European Society of Cardiology. *Position statement of the ESC Council on hypertension on ACE-inhibitors and angiotensin receptor blockers*. 2020; https://www.escardio.org/Councils/Council-on-Hypertension-(CHT)/News/position-statement-of-the-esc-council-on-hypertension-on-ace-inhibitors-and-ang.

Index

Page numbers followed by "*f*" indicate figures, "*t*" indicate tables, and "*b*" indicate boxes.